HOW TO PLAY
YOUR BEST GOLF

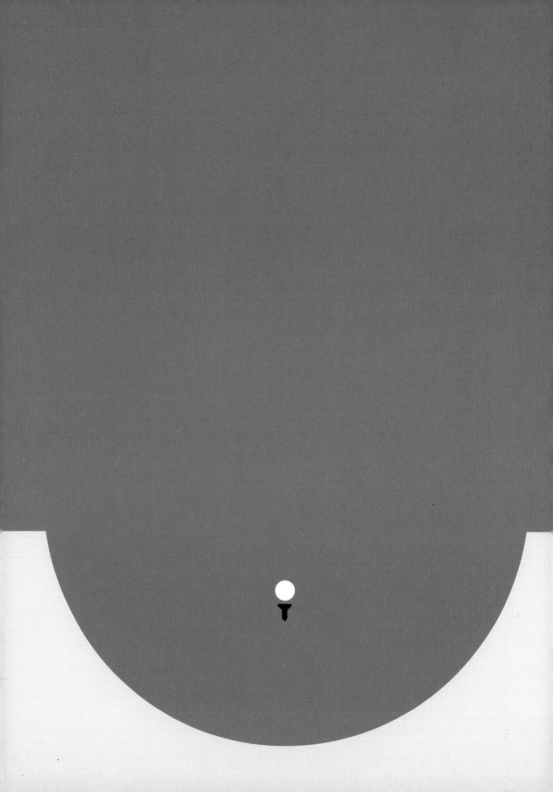

HOW TO
PLAY YOUR BEST
GOLF

Strategies From
a Tour Pro

NICK O'HERN

Hardie Grant

BOOKS

Contents

Part 3 Mental 122

Part 4 The Scoring Clubs 148

Part 5 A Game Like No Other 208

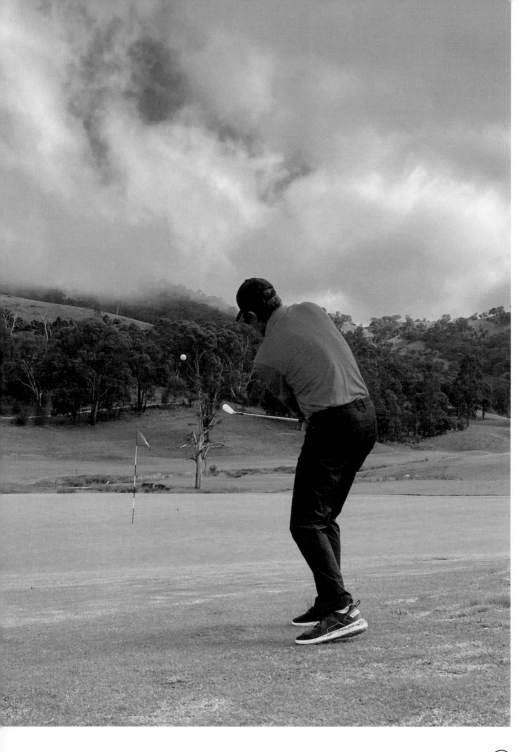

Preface

Since writing *Tour Mentality: Inside the Mind of a Tour Pro* in 2016, I've had some heartwarming feedback from a range of golfers on how it simplified a somewhat confusing and frustrating side of golf – the mental game. Perhaps reading something from a tour pro's point of view highlights the fact we all go through the same challenges, no matter our standard.

An interesting truth dawned on me recently; perhaps I'd known it all along and had just taken it for granted. The simplest way to shoot lower scores is by managing your way around the course in the most effective way that works for you. Sure, technique is important, but there are plenty of technically gifted golfers who can't post a decent score. Figuring out how to go around a golf course in the least strokes possible – that's the magic ingredient.

If I caddied for an 18-handicapper, their scores would drop by at least half a dozen strokes: a couple of shots from club selection, a couple from course management and probably a couple from simply reading putts. The good news is you don't have to change much with your physical game to lower your score. Like a signature, your swing and putting stroke are your own. Yes, there are certain fundamentals to follow, but I'm not here to tell you what position to be in at the top of your backswing. That's for the teaching pros of the world. Recently I helped a friend drop his handicap from 14 to 9 without even touching his swing. Instead, I showed him how to get the ball in the hole in the fewest strokes possible for his skill set.

Obviously there are various challenges with golf, but a couple stand out to me. Firstly, the game changes every time we tee up. During those four or so hours, different scenarios are encountered from round to round. It's inevitable, given golf's an all-weather game on an ever-changing playing field. It's why being flexible in our approach and continually adjusting to each situation is so important. Secondly, the ball is stationary. Most other sports have a moving ball, meaning you rely more on instinct and reacting. Golf is the opposite. You create the ball's movement – and have plenty of time to think about where it might end up.

The gap between the games that tour pros and the average golfer play is becoming wider than ever. Mostly this has to do with technology and how far tour pros hit the ball, and I'll get into that shortly. However, the principles for strategy, scoring and preparation apply the same to golfers all across the board. What saves half a shot for a tour pro is about the equivalent of five to six shots for a 20-handicapper. The secret is knowing what to look for, then moulding and adapting this information for your game. The following pages are a guide for exactly this, containing knowledge and insights I've accumulated over many years playing at the highest level, along with observing firsthand how the greats of the game go about their craft.

Enjoy the read and think well!

Cheers,
Nick

P.S. When referencing technique throughout the book, it's always from a right-hander's perspective. Even though I'm a lefty myself, the vast majority have yet to figure out the 'right' way to play the game. To keep things simple, I've bowed to the masses. ☺

P.P.S. This book is for golfers of all levels. From the tour pro through to once-a-month players at the local public course. Your skill set determines what you'll be able to do execution-wise for some of the different strategies and shots. If you can't hit a high draw 3-iron, that's okay – neither can I! Apply this information to what you do have and lower scores will follow.

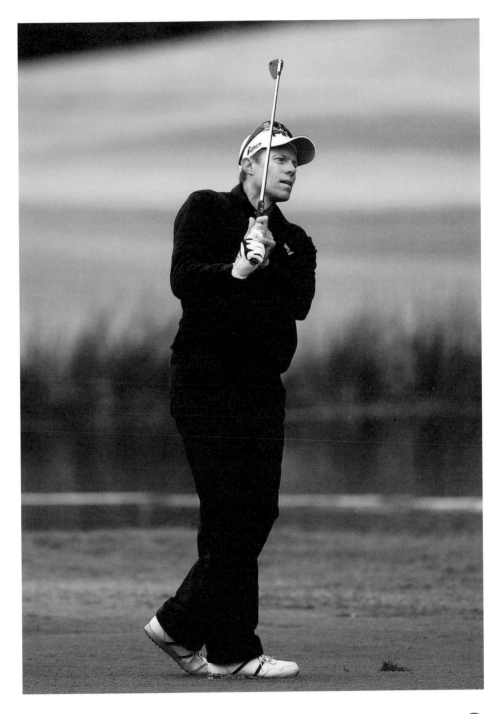

Introduction

'FORE!' Shouts echoed around the 13th tee at Royal Birkdale as Jordan Spieth watched his drive sail way to the right. It was the final round of the 2017 Open Championship and after 12 holes, Spieth was tied for the lead with playing partner Matt Kuchar. Starting the day with a 3-shot lead over 'Kuch', he'd given it all back over the front 9 after scraping and gouging his way around in 37, 3 over par. Kuchar, meanwhile, had played the same stretch in his customary consistent fashion for a level-par 34.

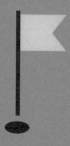

Pars on 10, 11 and 12 seemed to steady Spieth's wobbly ship. Then, on the par-four 13th, he hit his widest tee shot all week, some 50 yards (46 metres) right of target. His ball came to rest on the side of a dune under a gorse bush – unplayable. The only viable option for relief was a line-of-sight penalty that meant playing his next shot from the adjacent driving range. Determining where to drop was a monumental task in itself. Chaos reigned as spectators, rules officials and media all seemed to have their say in what to do next. In all, 17 minutes passed before Spieth hit his third shot over the dunes toward the green. His caddy, Michael Greller, did an outstanding job gathering all the necessary information regarding the line, distance, club and, more importantly, helping Jordan keep his composure throughout the entire ordeal. In the end, he holed a 6-footer for one of the all-time great bogies.

After spraying a shot that far off line, it's easy to assume he had no clue where the ball was going. Let's face it, we've all been there and thought, 'Get me to the clubhouse as quickly as possible.' Instead, Jordan walked off the green thinking, 'Wow, I can't believe I'm only one stroke back after all that!' It was an amazing escape and he felt like a stroke was gained rather than lost. Reinvigorated, he flushed a mid-iron to 4 feet on the par-three 14th,

resulting in birdie to draw him level with Kuchar again. On 15 and 16 he rolled in consecutive bombs going eagle-birdie, followed by a 12-footer on 17 for another birdie. It was mesmerising stuff and teeing off the 18th he had a 3-shot lead. A no-nonsense par four followed and the Claret Jug was his.

In the end, Spieth shot a one-under-par 69, and it's one of the most impressive rounds of golf I've ever seen. One under may not sound like anything special but, given the occasion and how it unfolded, to write this score down on the card was truly remarkable.

'Seventeen pars and a birdie would have been just fine,' he said later, 'but there's a lot of roads to get there.'

Jordan went through his entire golfing repertoire that day, the guile and cunning on display phenomenal. The emotional roller-coaster he went on exemplifies the challenges we all go through both physically and mentally during 18 holes. This game constantly toys with our emotions, providing stretches of both greatness and incompetence. I've played for more than 40 years and have learned one simple truth: golf is a continual problem-solving activity. At Royal Birkdale in 2017, Jordan was the best at it.

Part 1

Strategy

Play Like Your Personality

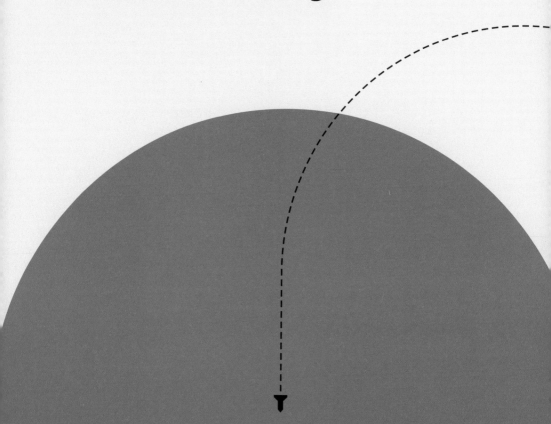

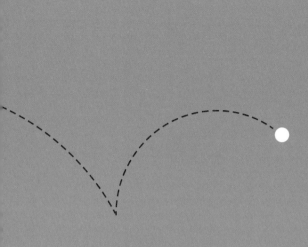

A common theme throughout this book is figuring out what works for you. Find your style of play, your brand, so to speak. There is no one way to play golf, and what works for me may not for you – or maybe it will. The important thing is to figure out what feels comfortable for you on the golf course and build your game around that. Here's a story with this in mind.

Pro-ams are part of every pro golfer's career at one point or another. When I was a young club pro starting out, they were a way for me to make a few dollars on the side while working in a pro shop. Then, after establishing myself on tour, the pro-am became a staple each week to thank tournament sponsors for their support. The tour event pro-am is the day before a tournament begins, and for amateurs it's a chance to play on the venue with a tour pro. Golf is unique in this sense – there's no other sport in the world where this occurs. Imagine playing a set of tennis with Roger Federer the day before a tennis tournament. Sorry, but it's never going to happen.

What continually fascinated me during pro-ams was how my amateur partners' games didn't reflect their personalities. Calm, relaxed people became incredibly nervous or angry and frustrated. Confident, gregarious types went quiet and seemed in a daze. I understand why: they were out of their comfort zone. On the first tee during a pro-am on the PGA Tour's West Coast swing, I looked over at my playing partner. There was a glazed look in his eyes and he was sweating, even though the weather was chilly. This guy was a heavy hitter in the business world but, at that moment, he was freaking out. I walked over, put my arm around his shoulder, smiled and said, 'Hey, just imagine doing this tomorrow.' He instantly laughed and let out the longest exhalation. 'I can't believe how nervous I am,' he said. 'I'm way out of my depth here.' My advice was simple: enjoy the day and play like you would with your mates.

It's easy to get caught up playing like someone else in stressful situations. Golf has a habit of making logic and reason simply disappear when you're out of your comfort zone. When this happens, self-awareness is the key to helping us realise things are spiralling out of control. From there we can direct our attention to the foundation for every shot on the course, the pre-shot routine (PSR). I'll review this in more detail later in Part 3: Mental, but applying your personality to the PSR, and your entire game for that matter, is a good starting point.

For instance, if you're more of an extrovert, it's actually a great idea to verbalise what you're about to do (although it can look a bit strange without a caddy!). It helps to get you involved with the process of the shot at hand. For an introvert, the opposite is true. It's okay to internalise things and go about your business as usual. For visual, creative types, seeing a shot in your mind beforehand is an invaluable tool to get you immersed in the shot. For analytical, data-driven types, gathering all the necessary information, computing the data and coming to your decision is crucial. There are various examples of these types of players. Lee Trevino, back in the day, was the epitome of a reactive player who made prompt decisions. He simply pictured the shot and reacted without hesitation. Currently, one of the fastest players on the PGA Tour is Matt Jones, and on the LPGA, Charley Hull. They trust their instincts, step up to the ball and execute. From an analytical standpoint, Jim Furyk, Bryson DeChambeau and Brittany Lang come to mind. They take their time to do the necessary due diligence and, when satisfied with the data and appropriate conclusion, move into the ball and execute. Some players also like to spend longer over the ball. Jack Nicklaus said he wouldn't pull the trigger until all unnecessary thoughts cleared from his mind. Personally, I can't do this, but obviously it worked for Jack. Of the current players, Jordan Spieth, Patrick Cantlay and Danielle Kang seem to fit this mould. All this brings up an interesting topic in golf – the pace of play.

Slow play has really become an issue. I find golf on TV is excruciating viewing at times, with players taking longer and longer to hit their shots, both on the men's and women's tours. Factoring in every possible calculation (especially on the greens with green-reading books) before pulling the club or deciding on a line seems to have become the norm. I'm all for taking in the necessary information for a shot, but part of the skill of playing golf is summing up a situation promptly. JB Holmes has driven plenty of viewers (and playing partners) mad with the amount of time he takes before shots, while Bryson DeChambeau wants to calculate every statistic scientifically possible, much to the chagrin of others. It works for them and, until rules officials bring in stricter measures for being slow, players will keep doing it.

As mentioned, it's important to find what works for you, but, please, if you can, do so without interfering with the pace of play. On tour, being known as a slow player is never a good tag because people just don't like playing with you. Fast players have to adjust to the slower ones, not the other way around. If you are on the slower side, one thing I'd suggest is to be ready to play when it's your turn. Don't wait for playing partners to hit and then start your calculations. Some of this can be done while they are playing their shot. That way, when it's your go, you're already well into the process of the shot. Don't spend too long over the ball. It allows negative and extraneous thoughts to infiltrate the mind.

Experiment with longer and shorter PSRs by thinking more and less too. Look at how long you spend over the ball – are you stationary or moving about before starting the swing? Go with what feels comfortable, as these are your natural tendencies – and when faced with a challenging situation, these tendencies become your safety blanket. This goes for every part of your game and relates in essence to whether you are more an artist, a scientist or somewhere in between. Once you understand what works and feels comfortable for you, the game of golf becomes simpler and your scores will follow suit.

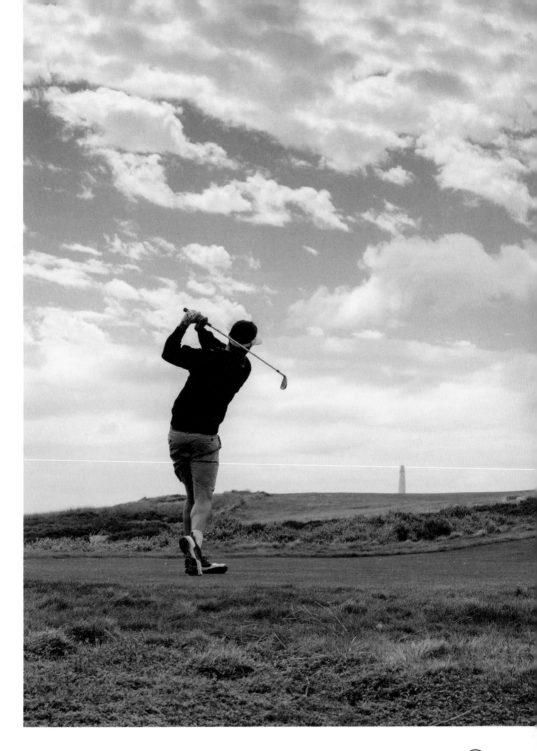

Play Like Your Personality

Course Management 101

The fastest (and simplest) way to shoot lower scores is through good course management. At the fundamental level, the following guidelines are a good template to work from. Obviously, varying conditions need to be considered for each shot, hole and course, but this is why being flexible in your approach to each situation is essential. Let's begin.

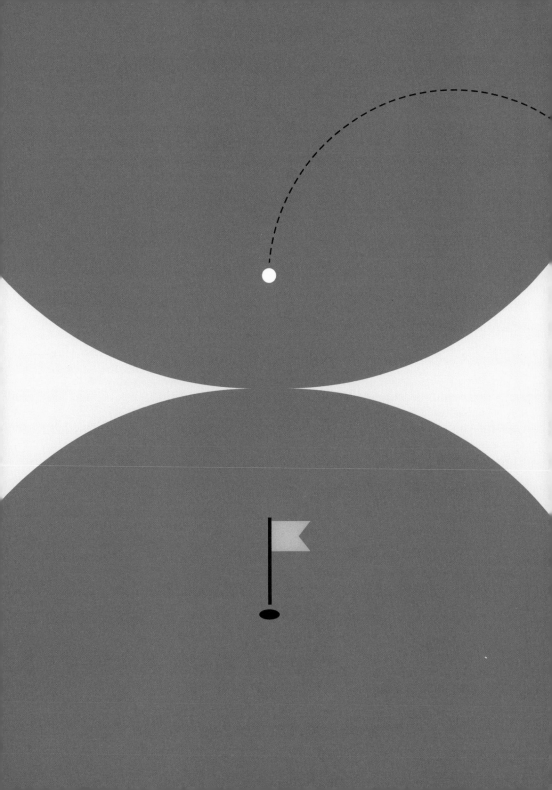

From the tee

USE THE TEE TO YOUR ADVANTAGE

Where you tee the ball up between the markers is important for the shot you want to hit. For example, on a dogleg left hole, ideally a right-to-left shaped shot is best suited. Teeing up on the left side opens up the right half of the fairway to shape the ball back into the centre. Conversely, for a dogleg right hole, the opposite is true. Tee it up on the right side, start the ball down the left and work the ball back from there. There are a couple of bonuses to this:

1. It gives the impression there's extra room to work with, providing more comfort from a mental standpoint thus freeing you up to make a good and confident swing.

2. If you start the ball up the correct side but without any shape, it finishes on the outside of the dogleg, a better position than too far on the inside. In most cases, the inside is where the danger lies on dogleg holes.

If, however, you can only hit one shape (for example, a left-to-right ball flight), then teeing it up somewhere in the right half of the teeing area will be more beneficial for you on just about every hole.

THE HOLE DETERMINES THE SHOT

I watched a great example of this during the final round of the 2020 USPGA Championship at TPC Harding Park in San Francisco. The 16th hole is a reachable par four with a slight dogleg right, and the Sunday pin was cut on the right side of the green hard up against a bunker. Overhanging cypress trees and gnarly rough down the right meant anywhere in that direction off the tee took birdie out of play. Left and long was the place to miss, if any. With all this in mind, the hole set up perfectly for a cut/fade driver to open up the front of the green to run the ball onto. Bunkers on the left side weren't ideal, but still okay, and further left was the Pacific Ocean, a definite no-no. I noticed several players trying to hit 3-wood to this narrow gap at the front, probably thinking driver was too much club. But it was the wrong shape for the hole because a full 3-wood for these guys typically means a draw. Five minutes after thinking this, Collin Morikawa stepped onto the tee, hit a perfect cut driver to 8 feet and rolled the putt in for an eagle two. It gave him a 2-shot lead, the eventual winning margin, and his first major at the age of 23. Talk about a wise head on young shoulders. Given his 2021 Open Championship win at Royal St Georges less than 12 months later, the sky's the limit for him.

Playing a hole based on how it's designed encourages a certain type of shot. Draw, fade, high, low and combinations of each. Your skill level and shot-making capabilities determine much of this and, in a way, modern technology has taken some of this finesse away. But think about certain holes at your course with this in mind: what's the right shot for this hole? If it's in your repertoire, great. And if not, that's okay, stick to what works. If you have the time and dedication, work on it at the range until you feel comfortable enough to take it out on the course.

USE THE WIND

Riding the wind enhances carry and roll from the tee. For example, on a right-to-left wind, a straight ball flight or a draw allows the ball to move in the same direction as the wind, assisting its journey. A left-to-right shape, however, balloons up against the wind and won't travel as far. The same goes for a left-to-right wind, but in reverse. Aiming down the left and either hitting a straight ball or a fade lets it ride the wind. A right-to-left shape fights it and gets knocked down out of the air too soon. Downwind, tee the ball right up and hit it high to use the wind for extra hang time. 'Tee it high, let it fly', as the saying goes. Facing into the wind, tee the ball lower to help keep it down out of the wind and use the ground to maximise yardage through roll. I'll detail how to hit these shots in a later chapter.

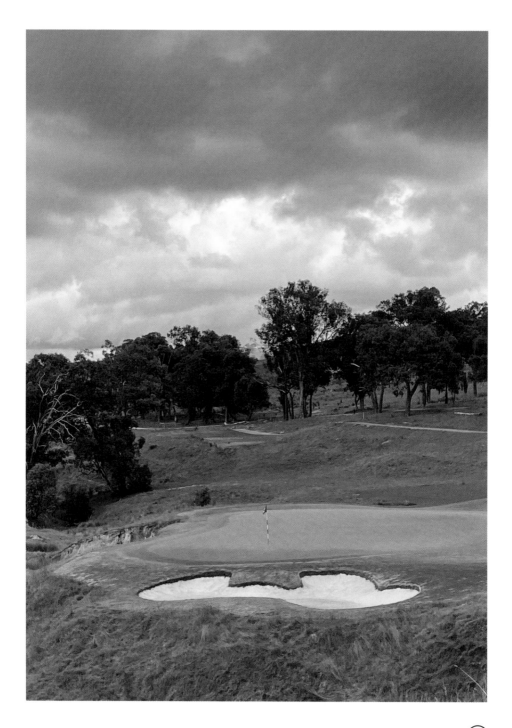

USE THE FAIRWAY SLOPE

I'm always looking to see if the tilt of a fairway can be used to my advantage. A couple that come to mind are the 10th hole at Augusta National and the 3rd hole on the East Course at Royal Melbourne. The 10th at Augusta is a sweeping downhill dogleg left par four with a steep slope running sharply from right to left in the landing zone. By working the ball with the slope (a right-to-left ball flight), it gets slung down the fairway for extra distance: always a good thing on this hole, given its length. The 3rd at Royal Melbourne East is a slightly different story. It's a downhill par four that doglegs right, and the entire fairway cambers that way. A lower ball flight up the left side allows the ground to do the rest for you. A higher trajectory brings in more trouble because the further down you go, the narrower it gets. Where distance isn't a factor, it's good to shape a ball against a severely sloping fairway to keep it in play rather than have it run off with the slope.

WORK FROM THE PIN BACKWARDS

A lot of holes (and courses) don't ask this question but the classic designs do. Standing on the tee my first thought is, 'Where's the pin position?' This determines the best portion of the green to hit the approach to, which answers where in the fairway is preferred to access this spot. Sometimes being in the rough on the correct side of a hole is better than being in the fairway up the wrong side. Great architects love to pose these questions on their courses. The Old Course at St Andrews and courses by Dr Alister MacKenzie (Royal Melbourne, Cypress Point, Augusta National), AW Tillinghast (Winged Foot) and Harry Colt (Sunningdale New) are some of the most enjoyable to play for this reason.

IT'S NOT ALWAYS DRIVER

On narrow holes, take a club you are confident of putting in play. It's better than trying to squeeze a driver down there, especially on shorter holes. If giving up some yardage off the tee isn't an issue, take a 3-wood or long iron/hybrid to keep the ball on the short grass. Hitting 8-iron into a green instead of wedge won't make that big a difference, and it's certainly preferable playing from the fairway than the rough.

Into the green

GET USED TO NOT AIMING AT THE PIN

Jack Nicklaus never went for the right-hand pin on the par-three 12th at Augusta National, and if his ball ended up there, it was a block. Even though it's only a short iron, Jack was content to play away from the pin on this dangerous hole and two-putt from distance. By going at sucker pins, you're tempting disaster, bringing in water hazards (in the case of Augusta's 12th hole) or areas very difficult to get up and down from. Short-siding yourself leads to double bogeys (and worse) if you get too cute with the recovery. The smart play is to the fat part of the green allowing some room for error. In general terms, for a right-hand pin, play left of the flag. A left-hand pin, right of it. A back pin, short of the hole, and a front pin, past it. There will be instances where these vary; however, what I'm getting at is you don't have to fire at every pin. By aiming away from the hole on the correct side, you have more room for error. For example, with a right-hand pin, if you aim left and you hit your intended target, you'll have a birdie putt of some length. If you pull it and miss the green left, then a par save is easier with plenty of green to work with. If you happen to block it, then you may even end up next to the hole ... like Jack but not on purpose.

WORK THE BALL INTO THE PIN

For a back-right pin I like to shape the ball in left to right from the middle of the green, so the ball's working toward the hole. The opposite is true for a back-left pin, by shaping it right to left. The key to these shots is:

a. you need the ability to shape the ball at will and, if so

b. favour the side of the green you are working the ball in from as your miss.

This way the ball is always moving toward the hole rather than away from it.

HOLD THE BALL AGAINST THE WIND

Opposite to riding the wind off the tee, you can increase the size of a green by holding shots up against a crosswind. For example, by drawing the ball up against a left-to-right wind, the ball lands softer and stops quicker, therefore the green becomes larger in area. If your ball rides the wind, a green's area shrinks because the ball releases more after landing, leaving less room to land and stop it in. Again, your skill level determines whether or not this is possible. There are variations though, based on pin position. For example, on a shot to a back-left pin with the wind out the right, by all means, use the wind to get the ball to that area. In golf, it's always situational.

PLAY TO THE BACK OF THE GREEN

Typically, mid- to high-handicap players believe they hit the ball further than they actually do. Try taking one extra club and play for the back of the green. More times than not, the middle or front of the green will be the result. Plus, with the thought of too much club, a smoother swing and a better strike will follow.

THE MIDDLE OF THE GREEN WON'T HURT YOU

This relates back to pin position. By playing to the middle of every green you'll never be too far from the hole and will usually be on the correct side. It's ideal when struggling with approach shots, especially on courses with very large putting surfaces. You may be quite a way from the hole, but at least you're putting. Hall of Fame legend Kathy Whitworth won 88 LPGA tournaments throughout her career (more than anyone on any major tour) and employed this strategy. You could say it worked for her. Golf is about minimising your mistakes; by aiming for the centre of every green, guess what: you avoid trouble more often.

OUT OF POSITION

Playing to the front or just short of the green is a wise strategy when you're out of position. Obviously it depends on what's around the front of the green, but typically being somewhere in front of the green provides a good chance to get the ball up and down. US Opens are a great example. Whenever I was in the rough, my first thought was to limit the damage by playing my next shot to an area I could make a score from (usually well short of the green leaving some sort of wedge in). A US Open is extreme in this regard, but it's important to weigh up the risk versus reward when you're not in an ideal spot. Scoring well is dictated by your decision from these areas, and the conservative option takes a big number out of play.

FACTOR IN BOUNCE AND SPIN

On firm greens, the bounce of a ball and its lack of spin need to be taken into account. For example, if you have 153 yards (140 metres) to the hole (and depending on how much spin you impart on the ball), your carry distance may be somewhere around 136–142 yards (125–130 metres), allowing for the ball to land, bounce and release. On softer greens, the total yardage is closer to the carry required, and sometimes even past the hole when balls are spinning back. For elite players, taking spin off of shots into soft greens is important with wedges and short irons. To do this, take one extra club and make a smooth three-quarter swing. This shot comes in very handy on windy days because it won't be affected as much by the wind. More on that later.

Around the green

IT'S NOT ALWAYS THE 60-DEGREE

Golfers love reaching for the lob wedge, and sure, sometimes it's called for (especially in the US where they grow rough up around the edges of greens), but often a less lofted club is a smarter play from cleaner lies. My strategy is to get the ball on the green as soon as possible (unless there are large slopes to negotiate) and let the ball roll the rest of the way. It simplifies shots because a less lofted club requires a shorter swing, meaning fewer things can go wrong.

LEARN THE FAIRWAY WOOD/HYBRID BUMP AND RUN

The bump and run is ideal for golfers who struggle with chipping, or when you have a less-than-perfect lie. A putter is useful, too, but can be difficult to swing hard enough from well off the green. A fairway wood or hybrid make it easier to achieve the required distance, plus they have more loft than a putter, elevating the ball through the first part of its journey to carry any rough patches. Experiment using these clubs from your chipping and putting set-up and grip. Personally, I prefer the chipping set-up and grip, but it's up to you. The ball comes off a little hotter than a putter, and with practice these shots can be game-changers for some. Tim Clark, the South African pro, was one of the best I've seen using these clubs around the greens.

TAKE YOUR MEDICINE

On short-sided shots it's important to be smart and not get too cute because, unless the shot is executed perfectly, it can lead to big numbers. There's no harm in playing for 10–20 feet past the hole and backing yourself to make the putt. At worst, you only drop one stroke. Short-sided means you're out of position and that comes with consequences. Don't make it snowball into something more than it needs to be. Now, if the lie's perfect and you feel comfortable, then by all means take it on.

Drill

Five clubs to one target: Find a spot around the practice chipping green, and chip balls with five different clubs to one target (hole). For example, lob wedge, gap wedge, pitching wedge, 9-iron and 8-iron. You quickly learn which clubs are best suited for the shot and which are higher risk. Then, either change the target (hole) or change position around the green for a different shot and repeat. It's fun to do this out on the course when no one's around.

On the green

OFFENCE OR DEFENCE?

Later, in Part 4: The Scoring Clubs, I'll talk more on green reading and the keys to great putting, but for now a couple of things to consider are the greens and the state of your putting. Firstly, are the greens fast, slow, smooth, bumpy, wet or severely sloped? A more defensive approach applies when they are either bumpy, extremely quick, severely sloped and/or when it's a windy day. Three-putts are more common, so instead focus on good speed and a more conservative approach for medium to longer putts. On slower, smoother and/or flatter greens, be more aggressive. It's easier to finish the ball closer to the hole, and even reducing the break is an option to give every putt a chance of going in.

Next, how you are putting needs to be taken into account. If you're struggling and have a downhill curling 15-footer, aim to finish the ball somewhere around the hole for, at worst, a tap-in rather than being aggressive and leaving a longer putt coming back. It's not a negative mindset, more a realistic one. However, if you feel like Ty Webb from *Caddyshack* holing putts at will, then by all means freewheel away and enjoy the zone. I played with Brandt Snedeker in the final round at Hilton Head 2011, where he lit the greens up. Every putt hit the back of the hole with speed and the look in his eye was enviable. Starting the day 6 shots back, Brandt shot 64 to force a playoff with Luke Donald, then won on the third extra hole – nanananana!

Course strategy

MAKE A PLAN

Review the course beforehand. See which holes present opportunities to attack, which are more suited to a conservative approach, and everything in between. Do it before you play – when your logic and reason are still intact. It's amazing how our thinking can change in competition, and we take on crazy shots. Tiger Woods's performance at Hoylake in the 2008 Open Championship was the result of executing a well thought-out plan. During practice rounds he discovered hitting irons from the tee was a more effective strategy. The fairways were bone dry and rolling out a long way, bringing into play the course's main danger – fairway bunkers. Advancing the ball out of them was minimal and, basically, they were a one-stroke penalty. Taking irons off the tee meant being short of these bunkers and further back but, importantly, in play. The ball-striking clinic he put on throughout the tournament confirmed his plan to be the correct one. As did the Claret Jug he held aloft at week's end.

PLAY TOUGH HOLES WITH LESS STRESS

For golfers with handicaps, playing a tough par four as a short par five takes away the anxiety you feel when playing the hole as a par four. Bogey is not the end of the world and if you get a stroke on the hole, it's a net par. This mindset allows you to play it more conservatively and with less stress. The same goes for difficult par threes and par fives.

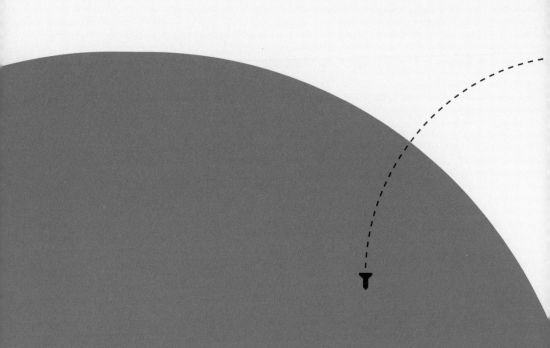

The Lure
of Distance

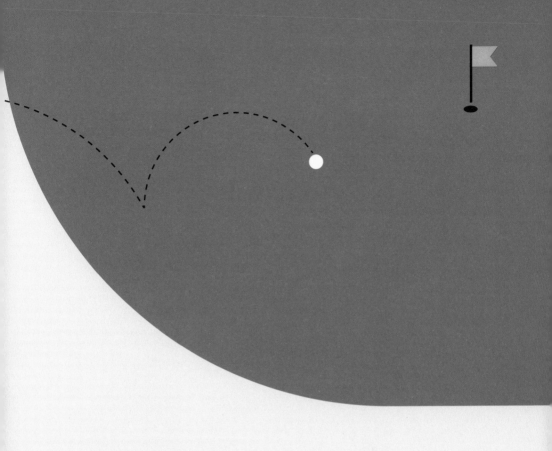

The game of golf has changed since my youth, but every sport evolves over time. It's only natural for us to keep coming up with new ways to improve. What were once thought unbreakable records have become the norm. The 10-second barrier in the 100 metres, the four-minute mile or throwing 100 mph fastballs to name a few. Popular thinking is that athletes are getting fitter, faster and stronger – but are they?

There's a fascinating TED Talk by David Epstein posing this question. As an example, he explained that in 1936 Jesse Owens held the world record time of 10.2 seconds in the 100-metre sprint. If Owens had raced in the 2013 World Championships, he would have finished 14 feet behind Usain Bolt's winning time of 9.77 seconds. Even though 0.43 of a second doesn't sound like a lot, in sprinting it's a chasm. But think about this: Bolt propelled himself from custom-made blocks and ran on a specially fabricated carpet designed for him (and everyone else) to run as fast as humanly possible. Owens ran on cinders (the ash from burnt wood), a much softer surface requiring more energy to run on. And rather than having a block to start from, Owens used a gardening trowel to dig holes in the cinders to put his feet in. Epstein points out that scientists have done biomechanical analysis of Owens's joints from the 1936 race and determined that if both runners had competed on the same surface, Owens would have finished within one stride of Bolt, or less than one-tenth of a second behind. I'm sure the shoes both wore made a difference too, but this wasn't accounted for. Epstein continues on to various examples in other sports, surmising the three determining factors when it comes to advancements in human performance throughout history in sport: genes, mindset and technology.

Genes relates to specific body types being more suited to different sports. For example, Michael Phelps is one of the greatest swimmers of all time and is 6 foot 4 inches tall (193 centimetres). Hicham El Guerrouj is a middle-distance runner who still holds the world record in the mile and stands 5 foot 9 (176 centimetres). There's a 7-inch difference in height, yet both have the same length legs. In swimming the ideal body type is a longer torso and shorter legs. In running it's the opposite.

Mindset is an area that athletes are continually improving by pushing boundaries – through both how they train and how they understand the mind regarding peak performance. Before Sir Roger Bannister broke the four-minute mile in 1954, everyone thought the elusive sub-four minutes was unattainable. Forty-six days after Bannister did it in 3 minutes 59.4 seconds, John Landy broke the record running 3 minutes 58 seconds. One year after Bannister broke four minutes, three athletes ran under the mark in the same race! Believing it could be done was the first step, and ultimately this opened the floodgates.

Technology is the third and largest cause of advancements in golfing performance, especially in recent years. Put simply, technology has altered the way players approach the game. Yes, fitness has played a part, but there have always been great athletes throughout the game's history. The ball and driver, however, have had the biggest impact, with two dramatic shifts occurring in the past few decades. Firstly, in the mid-90s metal woods began appearing, and slowly but surely the size of the driver head increased. Then in 2001 came the introduction of a three-piece ball as opposed to the wound version. The resulting gains in distance are from a combination of both improvements but, for me, the driver may have had the bigger impact.

I grew up using persimmon woods, which were incredibly difficult to control unless you found the middle of the clubface. Thus, a smoother swing for consistency, rather than power, was taught. Currently, with oversized driver heads and the forgiveness they allow, the approach has changed to 'hit the ball as hard as possible and figure the rest out later'. This philosophy is ideally taught during childhood, when clubhead speed gets locked in for the rest of a golfer's playing days. Making these increases is tougher the older you get, although Bryson DeChambeau has shown it's possible – but 99.9 per cent of golfers aren't going to follow his example of bulking up in the gym. Coupled with that though, he also studied and implemented the power moves (to some extent) used by long-drive champions. Only time will tell how long Bryson's body holds up, but his success already has younger players looking to add body weight and train harder to gain as much power in their games as possible. And they have to because length is such a factor in professional golf now. It's the obvious way to gain an advantage, and technology allows them to do so because if you miss-hit the ball with today's drivers, the ball still goes relatively straight.

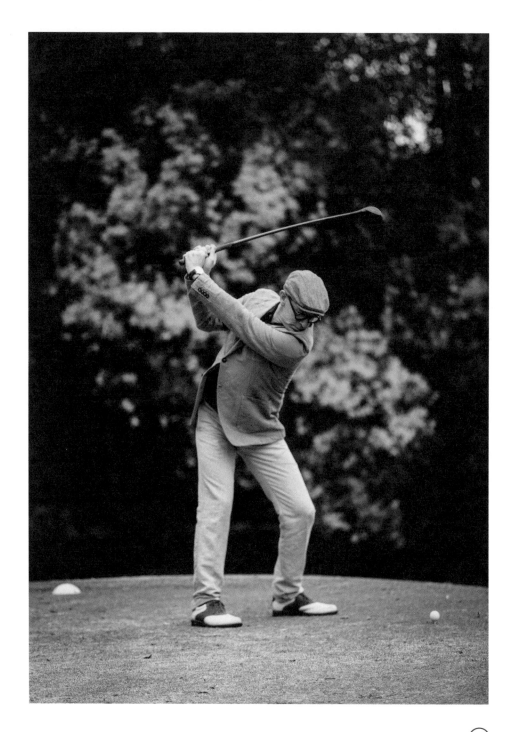

The majority of current-day players have been influenced in some way by Tiger Woods. Bursting onto the scene in 1996, Tiger's sheer athleticism and style of play signalled a new era. His impact, combined with advances in equipment, video, data and fitness, have made for a potent cocktail of power. After crushing the field in the 1997 Masters at Augusta National, the knee-jerk reaction of tournament venues was to lengthen their courses. The trend has unfortunately continued ever since. Tiger's dad once said if you want to 'Tiger-proof' a course, make it shorter, not longer. Lengthening a course only gives him (and longer hitters) more of an advantage. Shortening it levels the playing field, bringing position, shot-making and craft back into the equation.

Long hitters have always been around, but they were rare. Bobby Jones, Sam Snead, Jack Nicklaus and Greg Norman on the men's side, with Babe Didrikson Zaharias and Dame Laura Davies on the ladies. At the elite level now, distance has become a necessity in the men's game and it's becoming more so for the women too. In 1997 the PGA Tour average for driving distance was 267 yards (244 metres). John Daly topped the list with an average of 302 yards (276 metres), the first time the 300-yard barrier had been broken. In 2018, 296 yards (270 metres) was the average, with Rory McIlroy leading the way with 320 yards (292 metres), while 58 players averaged over 300 yards off the tee. On the European Tour the average was 294 yards (269 metres), Ryan Fox topped it at 321 yards (293 metres), and 62 players averaged over 300 yards (274 metres). On the Korn Ferry Tour (KFT), Cameron Champ averaged 343 yards (314 metres), while 101 players averaged over the 300 mark. That last number is the scariest because KFT players are the next generation coming through. I actually found the KFT tougher than the PGA Tour. In consecutive tournaments I shot 5-under and 6-under after two days and missed both cuts. Sure, the courses weren't as hard, but those guys make golf look like a pitch and putt, and they're coming in droves.

In a way, there are two games being played at the moment. One by tour pros and elite amateurs (e.g. college players), and another by everyone else who plays golf for fun and a bit of competition. The latter make up the vast majority of golfers, so I'm all for bifurcation of the rules, much like in baseball. Professional baseball players use wooden bats, while amateurs use the aluminium variety. This solves the issue of changing all the historic stadiums and ballparks to accommodate the power that technology would bring along with it. Imagine if they changed Wrigley Field in Chicago or Fenway in Boston. It sounds, and is, ridiculous. But in golf this is what we are having to do with some of the great courses because they're in danger of becoming obsolete otherwise. Lengthening them has been the natural reaction, but where does it stop? We could easily maintain the integrity of great courses by introducing a ball that's more difficult to control (make it spin more) and reducing the size of the driver for professional golf tournaments. I'm not saying let's go back to persimmon, but perhaps make the maximum head size 300 cc. Watching Greg Norman smash a balata ball with a persimmon head down the middle was something to behold and incredibly unique. Now, long, straight hitters are a dime a dozen. Long driving won't disappear, but long, *straight* driving will become a skill again because at the moment the driver is the easiest club in the bag to hit, whereas it used to be the hardest. For everyone else, let them use current technology. Elite amateurs will convert over to the pro ball and driver, so that they're accustomed when making the switch to pro ranks. The same happens in baseball for college and elite ball players. Time will tell what the United States Golf Association (USGA) and The Royal & Ancient Golf Club of St Andrews (R&A) come up with – pressure is mounting in this regard.

Interestingly, distance is magnified for golfers with higher swing speeds. The faster a person swings the club the greater the gain. For example, if I increased my swing speed from 100 mph to 105 mph, the gain in distance would be around 10 yards (9 metres). If someone with a swing speed of 115 mph increased it to 120 mph, they would gain 25 yards (23 metres). It's the same increase in speed yet a much higher gain in distance. So, in a way, the longer hitters are distancing themselves from the shorter hitters even more, and it's occurring in both the men's and women's games. Players such as María Fassi, Anne van Dam, Bianca Pagdanganan and Patty Tavatanakit have really started upping the ante on the LPGA in this regard.

Being more a feel player, I never knew all the different numbers, such as clubhead speed, spin rate and smash factor, when I was playing full-time. Driving-distance stats were always published so I knew those (I averaged between 260–270 yards /#238–247 metres my entire career), but using a TrackMan or other measurement device was never of interest – in hindsight, maybe to my detriment. I've been with Ping my whole career and the reps on tour would give me the latest drivers and shafts to try every so often to see if there was a benefit in changing to the newer model. After a couple of hits, I'd tell them yes or no completely by feel. 'Not sure what the numbers are, but this one's perfect,' I'd say. They'd take some readings, inevitably come back and say, 'Yep they're perfect.' Apparently, I was their lowest-maintenance guy on tour – lol. Using technology and data can be of great benefit in helping golfers with their games, but just remember to be careful. I've seen a number of players go too far down that rabbit hole and end up becoming driving-range players rather than golf-course players.

My intent here isn't to argue or debate what's correct distance-wise, more to explain that for the vast majority of golfers (those not aspiring to play for a living) it's not the be-all and end-all. People often ask me why I didn't try to hit the ball further. I found the harder I swung the worse things got, so I quickly realised playing my game was the best way forward. This involved hitting the ball straight, a good short game, and thinking well. When my putter was hot, I'd be on the leaderboard. This style of play led to me being a very consistent player for a number of years but not streaky enough to win many tournaments. I had plenty of top 10s, but victories? I can count those on one hand. My lack of length was, however, an advantage in match play because I hit approach shots into par fours and fives before my opponent. It enabled me to apply pressure on them after I knocked my ball in close. It was part of my strategy and a key ingredient to the success I had in the format.

Distance-wise I represent the larger population of golfers, and my thinking is if you want to hit a 7-iron further, use a 6-iron. As simple as it sounds, it's a great mindset for the course. The only club to consider hitting further is the driver. Given the size of heads now, yes, you can stand there and wail away, but beware. If you try to hit them too hard, the rough may be visited more than the fairway. At the pro level this isn't such a big deal because statistics* are showing players that being in the rough, and far enough down, is better than being in the fairway and much further back – Bryson DeChambeau's strategy at Winged Foot during the 2020 US Open being a prime example. Crazy as it seems, it's happening. For the average golfer this particular strategy doesn't work as well because their recovery skills aren't up to that of a tour pro, causing more damage to the scorecard than they would by playing a more consistent game. And the one thing people always ask me is, 'How can I be more consistent?'

A high percentage of poor shots for most golfers come from miss-hits through trying to hit the ball too hard. The perfect 7-iron that flew 164 yards (150 metres) and stopped right next to the hole from years ago is all they remember. I'm all for recounting great shots, but how often do they actually hit a 7-iron 164 yards through the air? Maybe two out of 10 tries. A more beneficial approach is to take 6-iron and focus on a nice smooth swing, thereby improving the chances of solid contact dramatically. With plenty of club, the focus shifts to rhythm rather than smashing the ball 5–10 yards (4.5–9 metres) further. Here's an interesting experiment to try: play 9 or 18 holes and take a club you think will get to the back edge of every green. At the end of the round see how many made it there or went long, and how many ended up in the middle or front half of the green. The ratio should give you a good indication for club selection. It's only natural to think you hit the ball further than you actually do and, yes, a 7-iron may travel 164 yards (150 metres) once in a while. However, if you only tried to hit it 153 yards (140 metres) your consistency will improve and so too greens in regulation. For elite players who regularly hit shots to specific numbers, this probably isn't a game for you, unless you like downhill putts from the back of greens.

---

*DECADE Golf is a statistics platform providing information for golfers on strategy regarding percentages and odds of playing from certain areas and distances. In a way it's like the Moneyball of golf.

My recommendation is this: work with your local PGA teaching pro to get the most out of the driver. There are different ideas regarding this, but I fall into the old-school method of not restricting the hip turn on the backswing and thereby lifting the left heel. Studies have proven that the average golfer can gain 5 mph clubhead speed simply by doing this. Brandel Chamblee talks in depth about these points and more in his book, *The Anatomy of Greatness*. He's done a lot of research in this area and it's well worth the read. For the rest of your clubs, focus on control over distance. Taking one more club is not the end of the world, and it will give you the consistency you're looking for.

The Lie
Dictates
Everything

During my last couple of years in the US before moving back to Australia, I coached and mentored several golfers, spending more time with one young pro in particular, Austen Truslow. His parents contacted me after reading *Tour Mentality* to see if I'd be interested in helping him. As a 17-year-old, Austen was the No. 2 player in the country but subsequently struggled through college and lost his way a little. During our first session together, I was immediately struck by the quality of his ball striking. He worked with renowned golf coach Mike Bender and his swing was technically outstanding. Ball striking—wise, it was as good as it gets, and I've seen some of the best. Being great on the range, however, doesn't mean you'll be a great player. Golf is about solving problems and adapting to a variety of situations. Every shot on the course is different, unique. So, building a repeatable, mechanical swing is an interesting proposition when golf asks you to do otherwise.

When working with a new player, I like to play with or watch them in a competition early on. Observing someone in practice and in a tournament are two completely separate things. In Austen's case we played a Moonlight event (a Central Florida mini tour) together at a course that wasn't in the best condition, but it turned out to be the perfect canvas to get an early message across. He shot level-par 72, while I shot 67. After the round he paid me one of the funniest compliments I'd ever heard. 'That was the un-sexiest 5-under I've ever seen,' he said. Once I stopped laughing, I replied, 'Thanks. By the way you should have shot 9 under.' He looked stunned.

So, I went back over his round and explained what could have been done differently. Austen's ball striking was superior to mine but, as our scores showed, that's only a piece of the scoring puzzle. The good news was his willingness to learn and his admirable work ethic meant we made some great strides in his game. It's going to be fun seeing how far he goes in professional golf. At the time of writing he's on the Korn Ferry Tour and progressing well. There is one fascinating quirk to his game – he chips one-handed. It works for him and that's all that matters. I looked at changing him to chipping with two hands, but after a while we realised his ball striking is that good, he doesn't need to be great at chipping. And, if you didn't watch him hit a chip shot and only followed the ball you'd say, 'Yep, this guy's good at chipping!'

Throughout our on-course sessions, something I continually impressed on Austen was the importance of how the ball lies – in the fairway, the rough, in bunkers and so on. Eventually he said, 'You could write a book on just this.' I'm not sure about that, but it's no coincidence this is one of the longer chapters because, quite simply, the lie dictates everything. It has the largest influence on what type of shot you're able to play. The only perfect lie on the course is when we tee off or putt on the green. Apart from those, there's always something to take into account in relation to how the ball reacts off the clubface. The subtleties can be almost unnoticeable but make a world of difference. In this chapter I'll be talking about lies for full shots. We'll delve into lies closer to the green in the short game chapter (page 186) later on.

From the rough

The rough affects the lie more than anywhere else on the course, offering a variety of things to consider, including type and density of grass, sandy areas, hardpan, pine needles and moisture.

LONG GRASS

Firstly, look at the way the grass is lying: with or against you. When it lies in the same direction you're going, the ball comes out better than when it's against you. Take this into account for club selection. Longer and/or thicker grass tends to wrap around the hosel of the clubhead, causing it to twist shut in your hands through impact. To prevent this, increase your grip pressure for a firmer grasp. Also, a less lofted club can lead to smothered shots and the ball staying in the rough. If in doubt take more loft, put the ball back in play and go from there.

A priority in the rough is getting the clubface on the back of the ball as soon as possible, and a steeper angle of attack helps with this. Too shallow (a normal swing), and the club has to travel through more grass to reach the ball, affecting contact. To come in steeper, either move the ball back in your stance a little, or lean your weight into your front leg slightly, or both on more severe lies. Then, pick the club up sharper by hinging your wrists earlier in the backswing, which also promotes a steeper angle of attack. Hybrids can be very handy clubs too because their wider surface area on the sole glides through the rough easier.

FLYERS

These occur when grass comes between the ball and clubface at impact, filling the grooves. The ball comes out with little to no spin, flying further than normal. Flyers are more common in lighter, wispy rough, whereas thicker, denser rough has a deadening effect. Bermuda is probably the strain of grass that prompts flyers most. The harder you hit the ball from a flyer lie, the hotter it comes out, and it's tough to control how far they go. The best option is to take one less club (8-iron instead of 7-iron) and swing away as per normal. It's a best guess, but this should be close to equalling things out distance-wise. Sometimes it may mean taking two less clubs, especially if short of the green is better than long. Another option is taking the club you'd normally use and putting a smooth three-quarter swing on the ball. Also, factor in that the ball will release more when it lands through lack of spin.

WET ROUGH

The ball comes out softer because moisture accumulates in the grooves between the clubface and the ball. This has a deadening affect, so taking an extra club (7-iron instead of 8) is worth considering.

SANDY LIES

How firm or soft the ground or sand is determines your options. Off a baked, hardpan lie, it's easy to catch the ball thin, since the club can bounce off the ground. Play it slightly further back in the stance for a cleaner strike. From softer lies take a good look at how the ball's lying. Slightly down in the sand means solid contact will be difficult, so take your medicine and get the ball back in play. Don't compound the mistake you already made from being in there.

PINE NEEDLES

Two things to factor in are:

1. They are slippery to swing in. To prevent sliding about, create a solid stance at set-up, take an extra club and make a smooth three-quarter swing.

2. The ball won't curve as much. If pine needles are gathered around the ball and you can't get a clean strike on it, the ball slides up the clubface through impact, rather than being compressed.

When the ball's lying clean, it's easier to hit a draw than a fade. A couple of memorable shots have been struck at Augusta National during The Masters, where pine needles (or pine straw as it's called in the US) cover the rough all over the course. In a playoff during the 2012 Masters, Bubba Watson famously hooked a wedge from pine straw deep in the trees on the 10th, which led him to victory. Being a lefty definitely helped because a right-hander wouldn't have been able to curve it that much with a slice. Even so, the amount of shape he imparted on the ball was ridiculous.

In the final round of the 2010 Masters, Phil Mickelson's 6-iron second shot on the par-five 13th off the pine straw was one for the ages. With the tournament on the line, he gambled by going for the green, even though later on he called it the percentage play. Everyone else thought he was crazy, and it looked a pretty hard sell to convince his caddy, Jim 'Bones' Mackay. I think Bones even considered using his veto* there. Phil made the right decision. He nailed the 6-iron between two trees, carried the creek at the front by a yard, and ended up 4 feet from the hole. He missed the putt for eagle, but the resulting birdie gave him the necessary momentum to claim his third green jacket.

---

*Phil Mickelson's former caddy, Bones, got a veto once a year to override a shot he thought Phil had absolutely zero chance of pulling off. A famous non-veto occurred in the 2002 British Open at Muirfield when Mickelson's ball came to rest just in the right-hand side of a fairway bunker. As a left-hander, he had no shot and wanted to hit a 6-iron off his knees from outside the bunker. Bones tried to exercise his veto, but Mickelson said they were for domestic use only and didn't count overseas. Bones filed a grievance, which fell on deaf ears, since Mickelson was the veto commissioner. He proceeded to hit the ball two fairways away and ended up making a 20-footer for a triple bogey seven. I think Bones might have had a valid argument.

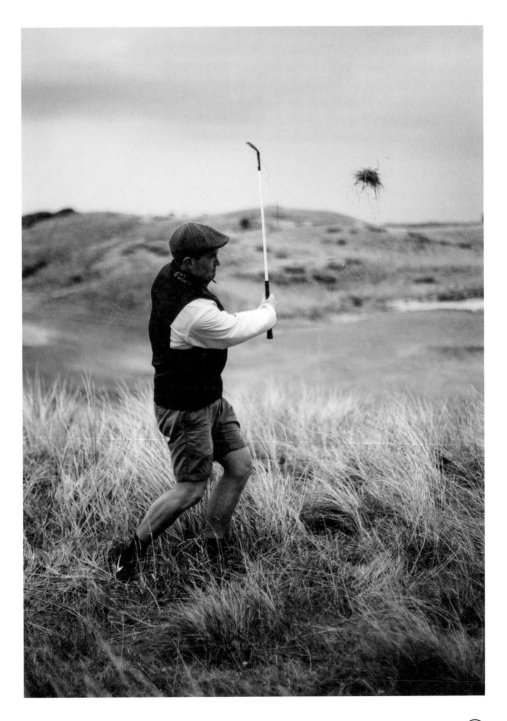

The Lie Dictates Everything

'Riviera Country Club in Los Angeles is one of the most famous courses with kikuyu fairways. You don't get much roll off the tee, but it's lovely to play off.'

In the fairway

Hitting the fairway should mean a nice lie, right? Well, golf can be cruel – that doesn't always happen.

TYPE OF GRASS

I grew up playing on couch fairways in Perth, and many of the Melbourne sandbelt courses have this variety too. During summer, they become very firm and it feels like you're hitting off concrete at times. During the Australian Masters at Huntingdale back in 2005, my playing partner, the aforementioned Bubba Watson, found this out firsthand. He attacked the ball so steeply with his irons, he resorted to letting go of the club straight after impact because it jarred his hands so much. But, like all top players, he still found a way, and finished second in the tournament. Links courses in the UK have very firm fairways made up mostly of fescue grass, which does well in cool climates and coastal regions. In general, playing firmer fairways requires a shallower** swing, otherwise your teeth can hurt from the jarring.

Conversely a soft, spongy grass like kikuyu has a much different feel. The ball sits up nicely and the grass's cushioning effect allows a more downward strike that creates extra spin, especially with the short irons. Riviera Country Club in Los Angeles is one of the most famous courses with kikuyu fairways. You don't get much roll off the tee, but it's lovely to play off. Bermuda is a softer variety too and found in humid climates, such as Queensland (Australia), Florida (USA) and various parts of Asia. It's one of the few grasses that can survive in hot conditions. Bermuda has a lot of grain, which must be accounted for. Down grain is easier to play off and has little effect, but, into the grain the clubface can grab and dig into the ground, leading to fat or chunked shots. Coming into the ball slightly steeper (which requires a little more precision) and/or taking one extra club with a smooth, three-quarter swing are a couple of good options if you're unsure with this lie.

POOR LIES

A ball sitting in a depression requires a slightly steeper angle of attack for solid contact. Shift the ball position back a touch, so your hands are just ahead of the clubface at address. For a ball in a divot, look at which part of the divot it's in. The back part requires a much steeper angle into the ball than if it's at the front or middle section. Bear in mind the ball will come out lower and has a tendency to squeeze right, so adjust accordingly.

**For a shallower swing, practise hitting shots from a slope with the ball above your feet. It helps to stay taller through the ball and has a shallowing-out effect. Another drill is to hit mid irons off a tee in the ground at driver height. The idea is to clip the ball off the tee rather than going underneath it. Focus on staying taller and maintaining width throughout the swing.

Sloped lies

One of the most common variations is playing from sloped, uneven lies. It happens in the fairway, from the rough, around the greens and in bunkers. Every golf course is different regarding how undulating they are. Even flat courses still have gentle slopes and cambers that are felt only when walking the fairways and standing over shots. I've also played courses so hilly that a flat lie is welcome relief. The Highercombe Golf Course, outside Adelaide in South Australia, comes to mind. After playing a few pro-ams there early on in my career, one leg felt longer than the other after a round. Miss-hits are the most common occurrence off sloping lies. For better contact, there are three key elements to keep in mind – set-up, alignment and club selection.

Regarding set-up, the one constant is a wider stance. How wide depends on the severity of the slope. A wider stance promotes stability and allows you to shift your weight around at set-up, so you can then align your shoulders appropriately, making it easier to swing with the slope. Exaggerate the wider stance to begin with, so you get an idea of how much stability you can create. In my experience, golfers don't widen their stances enough.

DOWNHILL LIES

With a wider stance, shift your weight into the left leg for balance and tilt your left shoulder lower so the shoulders feel in line with the slope. Keep your weight on the left side throughout the swing to help you swing down with the slope for solid contact. I like to walk out after the shot off downhill lies because it really gets me swinging down with the slope and through the ball. Gary Player was famous for doing this, even off flat lies. The most common miss-hit is a thinned shot from lifting up off the ball in an effort to get it airborne. From downhill lies the ball will fly lower and, if anything, go a little right, so aim a touch left to counter this.

UPHILL LIES

Again, widen the stance, but this time lower your right shoulder so it's well below your left and once again in line with the slope. This shifts your weight into your right leg and promotes the feeling of swinging up with the slope. Your swing will feel slightly restricted, especially in the lower body, so a three-quarter swing feel is ideal. Since shots tend to go left off this lie, aim right accordingly.

SIDEHILL LIES – BALL BELOW THE FEET

Widen the stance, flex the knees a touch more, and tilt your upper body from the waist a little extra to make getting down to the ball easier. The key is to stay in your posture throughout the swing. It's natural to come up out of the shot, leading to thinned shots. From this position the swing naturally becomes more upright and the ball usually veers right, so aim further left. How much depends on the severity of the slope.

SIDEHILL LIES – BALL ABOVE THE FEET

The feeling here is to be tall, with your upper body having less tilt than usual. The swing becomes more rounded, like a baseball-type action, helping prevent the club from digging into the slope. Typically, the ball moves left off these lies, so aim further right.

Sometimes you'll have combinations of the above. For example, a ball below the feet off a downhill lie. Stability is of numero-uno importance – building a solid base first is the key. Widen the stance, lean into your left side, align your shoulders, bend more from the waist and stay in this posture throughout the swing. Taking an extra practice swing or two beforehand helps you feel what the slope wants you to do. The focus is on solid contact, and with the right adjustments set-up-wise, it's very doable. Some practice doesn't hurt either. ☺

Regarding club selection for all the different slopes, a wider stance restricts the lower body, resulting in a slightly less than full swing. This is ideal for control and keeping your balance. Factor this in by taking an extra club on sidehill lies, and one or two extra clubs on uphill lies depending on how severe it is (because you are also adding loft by leaning back with the slope). On downhill lies you're delofting the clubface, which evens out the three-quarter swing effect, and on some downhill lies you'll take one less club. Remember, this is a guide. There will be circumstances where more or less club will be needed depending on the slope and conditions.

Fairway bunkers

Fairway bunker shots require staying centred and level throughout the swing for pure contact. Practising out of fairway bunkers is great for iron play in general because afterwards your strike improves immediately upon returning to the grass.

Mitchell Spearman, an English teaching pro based at Isleworth (my home club when I lived in Florida), once told me about a drill Nick Faldo did during his halcyon days. He'd hit 2-irons from a fairway bunker until striking them perfectly. It synced his swing up beautifully and, if not, showed up areas that required work. When I started this drill, what became apparent was everything after that felt like a piece of cake. I don't even use a 2-iron in tournaments (except on links courses) and long irons were never my strong suit. If I was able to hit these solidly, I knew my swing was on song and, if not, it's a 2-iron out of a fairway bunker for heck sake! Plus, after that my 4-iron looked like a 6-iron and was much easier to hit. It's a philosophy I build into all my practice sessions. Make part of it as difficult as possible, so the norm becomes easier.

Fairway bunkers (as with sloped lies) are about feeling stable, and staying level and centred. Dig your feet in when taking your stance for stability to prevent slipping (a slightly wider stance can help too). Since you're submerged in the sand gripping down the club a half inch or so is recommended. Personally, I grip these shots as per normal, but see what feels better for you.

Next, focus on a central point in your sternum to rotate around. This helps to stay centred and prevents moving up and down or side to side too much. Both lead to miss-hits. A little distance is lost out of fairway bunkers, so take an extra club (if the bunker lip height allows) and swing smoothly. The harder you swing the more chance there is of slipping and miss-hitting the ball.

CLUB SELECTION

Knowing what club gets over the lip is obviously important, and here's a simple way to figure this out: find a spot in a fairway bunker where, for example, a 6-iron feels comfortable to clear the lip. Hit a few balls and see if you are correct. If so, take a step closer to the lip and repeat. If you're still clearing it move closer, and closer, until you reach a point where a good shot catches the top of the lip. Move back a step and file that image in your memory bank. Change clubs and repeat. With solid contact you can actually use a less lofted club than you think. It just takes hitting balls to trust what you see. However, I do recommend erring on the side of caution by taking more loft to make sure you comfortably get the ball out.

SLOPED LIES

The same principles mentioned earlier apply. The advantage being you can dig your feet into the sand for more stability. Typically, not enough loft is taken from downhill or ball-below-the-feet lies, so don't bite off more than you can chew – take more loft. Firstly, you're in a fairway bunker and, secondly, it's not an ideal stance. Rather than the hero shot, get the ball to an area you can still make a score from. Too many scorecards are ruined trying to replicate the shot Tom Watson hit at Colonial in 1998 on the 9th hole. If you haven't seen it, take a look on YouTube, it's unbelievable!

POOR LIES

When the ball is sitting down in either a rake mark or in soft sand, contact has to be precise. In essence you're trying to pick the ball off cleanly, which feels like a slightly thinned shot and comes out lower. Near the lip, again err on the side of caution and take extra loft and, if anything, a slightly fat shot is the better miss. That way at least the ball comes out. From further back in the bunker thinned shots work well.

WET SAND

This is an easier proposition because moisture seals the top layer of sand, providing cleaner lies. After quite a bit of rain the sand gets compacted like hardpan. The only issue being that it's easier to slip on a hardpan lie, so dig the feet in!

WEDGES

Shorter clubs from fairway bunkers can be difficult for some, especially shots from closer range. The more loft, the more precise the strike needs to be, although being closer to the ball does help in this regard. An alternative for a shot of say 55–65 yards (50–60 metres) is to take a 7- or 8-iron and play it how you would for a regular greenside bunker shot with a full swing. From softer sand this can be a much higher percentage shot rather than trying to pick it clean with a wedge. Make sure you aim far enough left when doing this though, as the ball will squirt further right with an open-faced 7-iron than a sand wedge.

Yes, it takes practice

Getting comfortable with all the different lies and shots I've mentioned above takes practice, plain and simple. You'll need to think outside the box to find these lies because driving ranges are flat, and it's rare they have a fairway bunker next to them.

On the range, roll a ball onto the grass, rather than placing it, to practise poor lies in the fairway (depressions, divots and the like). We tend to put every ball on a perfect lie, and hence struggle with not-so-perfect ones on the course. Next, at the sides of the range (or front or back if it's quiet) usually there are areas with some slope and/or rough to hit from. Another option is the practice chipping green. Typically, there are slopes around it to hit balls off back onto the range.

When working on the above, exaggerate the key fundamentals: the wider stance, shifting your weight, coming in steeper. Overdoing these provides a better understanding of what's required. Having done so, you can always dial it back from there.

Finally, every time you walk up to your ball on the course, don't just reach for the laser straight away. Instead, take a look at the lie first and think about how it will affect the shot. Because I guarantee you, it will.

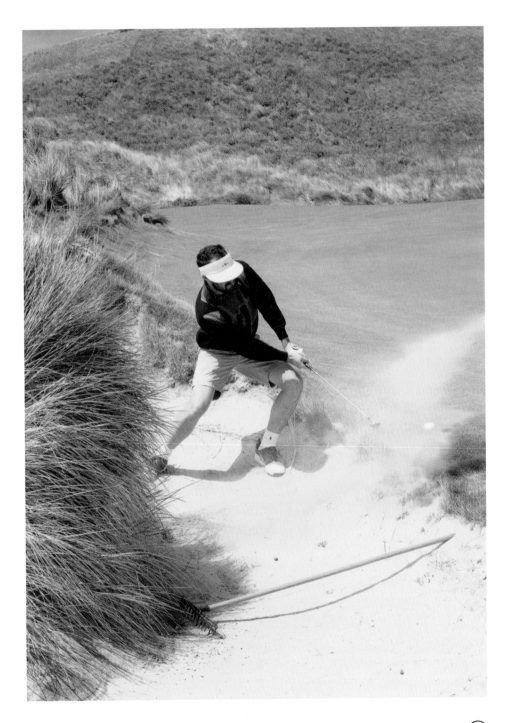

The Lie Dictates Everything

Pin High: The Shot Determines the Club, Not the Yardage

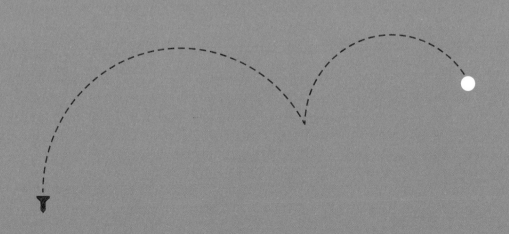

The importance of figuring out each shot as it presents itself cannot be overemphasised – which is why I will emphasise it repeatedly throughout this book. Part of solving these scenarios requires being analytical at times. However, the skill of being a golf-course player, rather than a driving-range player, lies in being creative, in seeing and feeling shots rather than just playing by numbers (yardages). Controlling distance and consistently being pin high is one of the most important elements to being a good golfer. It's what separates tour pros from everyone else. Finding the most suitable way to hit the ball the required distance has become somewhat of a lost art, especially in younger players now. But it's even happening in the old-school generation as well, mostly due to technology, in particular lasers.

A few years ago, I helped a fascinating guy in his late 50s named Richie Fulmer. Richie loves his golf, plays off a 2 handicap and regularly shoots in the 70s. During our first session, he explained how golf had become stale and frustrating. Certain shots were a struggle, namely trying to fade the ball. His natural shape was a draw and after observing him hit balls for a while, it became apparent he was a little too one dimensional, playing by numbers rather than what the shot called for.

To spark Richie's imagination, I asked him to hit shots to a target 135 yards (123 metres) away with five different clubs, starting with 9-iron, then 8-, 7-, 6- and 5-iron (the same 'five clubs to one target' drill on page 29). For him, 137 yards was a stock 8-iron, while every other club called for some feel and creativity, especially the 5- and 6-irons. I had him exaggerate a variety of trajectories and shapes with each club. Low fades, three-quarter bump and runs, baby draws and huge high cuts. All of a sudden, golf became fun and Richie's reaction was priceless. 'I haven't thought about hitting shots like these in years. I feel like a kid again,' he said excitedly. We went to the first tee to play 9 holes – with one condition. I said, 'When you arrive at the ball, rather than pulling out your laser and getting a yardage, figure out what shot feels right first. Then, if you want, get the yardage.'

It forced Richie to tap into the creativity he'd found on the range. His first reaction, however, was again to think in numbers. For his second shot on the 1st hole he said, 'Well, it looks like about 150 yards (135 metres) so that's my 7-iron.' I interjected, 'Don't think in terms of distance, more what shot and shape feel right, then relate that to a club.' In this case, the pin was back right, so a left-to-right flight was ideal. He pulled out 6-iron and hit a beautiful fade into the middle of the green, about 20 feet away. The lightbulb suddenly came on and he began visualising shots he hadn't considered in quite some time. After a few holes he even stopped lasering the yardage. It was one of the most enjoyable 9 holes I'd seen anyone play.

The lesson here is *the shot determines the club, not the yardage*. Or, as I like to say, there's never a wrong club, it just depends on the shot you want to hit. Let me explain.

My coach, Neil Simpson, told me a story about the time he played with the late great Kel Nagle at the Queanbeyan City Open (just outside Canberra) back in the late 70s. The 10th hole was an uphill par four and Neil's tee shot finished a couple of paces in front of Kel's in the fairway. As Kel got over his ball Neil thought, 'Geez that looks like a straight-faced club'. He didn't think too much of it and after both hit their shots, they walked up to the green. It turned out Kel had hit a 4-iron pin high, while Neil hit an 8-iron over the back of the green. He couldn't believe the disparity between the clubs and the shots. He realised Kel had seen a completely different shot to his own to get the ball pin high. How far he had or what club he 'should' use didn't matter. It was more about the shot Kel saw and, ultimately, believed in. It was an unforgettable lesson for Neil on the art of shot-making.

Great players have the ability to execute shots only they see and feel, without caring what anyone else thinks. Neil's story stuck with me throughout my playing career, so much so that I never took much notice of what club someone else used. It was usually a club or two less than me anyway, given my lack of length, so what was the point worrying about it? Plus, I'd get a kick out of knocking my longer iron closer than their shorter one. I find it amusing when players look in each other's bags to see what club the other's hitting. How can one person possibly know, firstly, what type of shot the other is going to hit, and, secondly, how they are feeling? Similarly, on the putting green if someone asks me what the line is, I say, 'It depends on your speed.' I don't know how hard someone's going to hit a putt because for me, speed determines the line (more on that later).

I love surprising players I help with a 'no yardages' game for 9 holes. They can't use their laser or look at distance markers, and they have to eyeball every shot playing purely by feel. 'How will I know what club to use?' they ask. 'See it and feel it,' I say. I'm amazed how many young golfers have never played a round of golf without yardages, and, admittedly, I get a sadistic pleasure taking that comfort away to see how they adjust. Sure enough, on the first hole they instinctively reach for the laser because it's become such a habit. I quickly put a stop to that and watch the struggle begin.

Initially, indecision kicks in because they're accustomed to relying on numbers. They haven't used their eyes and other senses to determine a shot, so club selection becomes an internal debate. This leads to poor swings because of doubt and they don't commit. After a while the realisation hits that it's better to be committed with the wrong club, than have the right one and be in two minds. At first, shots go long or come up short, but soon, their other senses come alive and their feel starts to improve. By the end of 9 holes, pin high becomes the norm. 'I don't know why I even need yardages,' some say. They come in handy, trust me, but golfers have gone too far down the scientific path and forgotten there's still an art to playing the game.

The biggest advantage of playing this way is when conditions are unique or quite tough, either from wind, rain, cold, heat, hard and fast and so on. For example, if the wind's blowing 40 km/h into you on a cold day, yardages don't mean a thing. You might be taking up to four clubs extra depending on the shot you want to hit. That's all based on feel, not numbers. I've played Open Championships in extreme winds where I've hit a 5-iron 120 yards (110 metres) on a hole, then on the next, in the opposite direction, hit 9-iron 197 yards (180 metres). It was so much fun!

I understand there are analytical golfers that need to play this way – a prime example being Bryson DeChambeau. But it's the feel players I love watching, like the late Seve Ballesteros back in the day, Lorena Ochoa before she retired and, currently Bubba Watson. Tiger Woods put on a clinic at Royal Melbourne at the 2019 Presidents Cup in this regard. The way he flighted the ball with different trajectories and shapes was a masterclass. I believe a blend of technical and creative elements is the best method. Which side the scales tip regarding this blend is up to the individual. I lean more toward the creative side. My caddy Wilbur (you'll hear from him later) knew not to give me a yardage until I asked for it. That way I could survey the situation first to get a sense for the correct shot and club. Then he'd give me the yardage to confirm my instincts.

Try the 'no yardages' game next time you play. Stand at your ball, look at the target and think, 'What shot feels right here?' Then ask yourself, 'What club is best suited to the shot I'm seeing?' Commit to that decision and swing away. Distance-wise you might be off to begin with, but it won't take long before you're consistently pin high. It's an enjoyable way to play, plus you'll expand your repertoire of shots in no time.

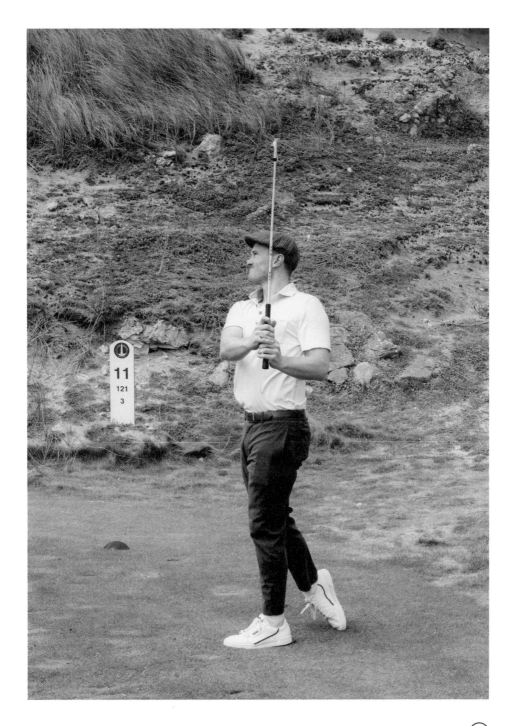

Pin High: The Shot Determines the Club, Not the Yardage

Know Your Strengths and Weaknesses

Zach Johnson's win at The Masters in 2007 was a David and Goliath moment in golf history, highlighted by the strategy he took on the long holes. Of the 16 par fives he played that week, Zach never went for a green in two. The par fives at Augusta National traditionally are where players make inroads on the scorecard, especially on the back 9 at the 13th and 15th holes. For him to win in this fashion was truly remarkable.

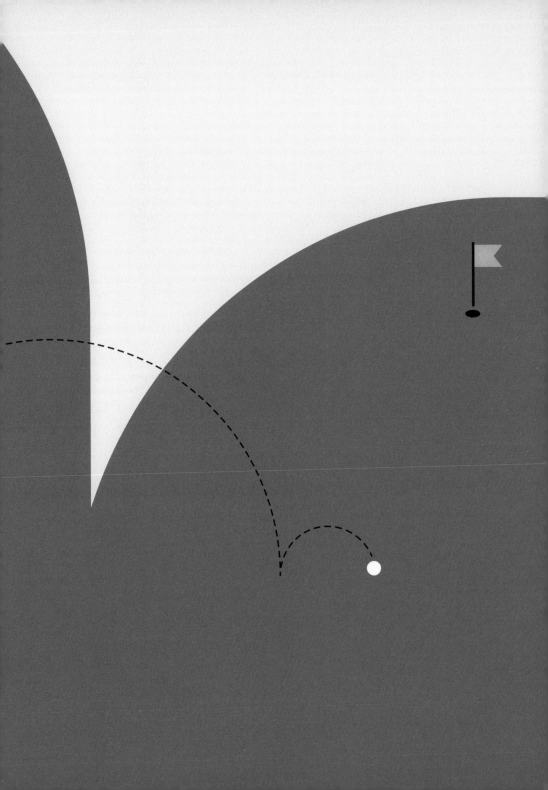

When Tiger Woods decimated the course in 1997 to win by 12 strokes, the Augusta National committee began the process of stretching the course out. Year after year, they added length to certain holes, and the fascinating part was the changes were virtually unnoticeable. I remember standing on the 11th tee in a practice round thinking, 'Hang on, I remember that tree being behind the tee, not in front of it.' Sure enough, the hole was 30 yards (27 metres) longer, yet it looked as though it had never been changed. Rather than simply moving the tee back they completely rebuilt the entire hill. With what seems like an unlimited budget, the Men of the Masters don't do shortcuts!

I was there (at least the first two days until I missed the cut) the year Zach won and remember the weather was uncharacteristically cold, turning an already long course into a monster. Zach's on the medium to short side lengthwise off the tee like me (although I'm just short), so in general the course doesn't present many opportunities to go low. But given the conditions this particular year, even more so. He obviously realised the chances of making eagle on the par fives by going for them in two was slim to none, so the best strategy was to play to his strengths – solid wedge play, putting well and sheer grit. This was never more evident than on the 13th hole during the final round. Tied for the lead, he faced a tantalising second shot that would have seen most players going for the green. Instead, he stuck to his game plan, laid up, wedged it close and made birdie. Two more birdies coming in on the 14th and 16th gave him a total score of +1 and his first major title, along with a stylish green jacket. By the way, on the par fives he was 11 under par for the week!

Discipline is the name of the game when sticking to a conservative game plan at Augusta National. Opportunities to gamble for a large gain continually present themselves. The downside being that the penalty is more severe than the reward in most cases. It's a great lesson for all golfers when playing a hole that's tempting you to hit a shot you shouldn't. Always play to your strengths and avoid your weaknesses.

Firstly, it's important to understand what both are. If you're not long off the tee, don't try to carry a fairway bunker at your limit. Instead play short of or around it, and rely on your iron play. If your short game is a weakness, aim for the middle of greens (a good strategy in general anyway) rather than attacking pins and leaving little room for error. Now, if you're a genius around the greens, by all means attack away. If hitting a draw is uncomfortable, perhaps trying to turn one around the corner on a dogleg left hole isn't the smartest idea. Stick to your stock shot and play the hole accordingly. These are just a few examples of how it's important to recognise what you can and can't do. Play within yourself, especially if you're unsure of the situation. Golf has a habit of presenting scenarios that show up weaknesses at critical moments. How we handle them determines our score for the day.

Practice-wise you'd think it's a no-brainer for golfers to work on their weaker points, but sometimes that isn't the case, even at pro level. I've seen plenty of great ball strikers, and that's mostly what they work on at the range – ball striking. They struggle to score because their wedge play and short game need more attention but get the least. They would improve simply by reversing their practice structure. A great exercise, for example, would be to practise with just the wedges and putter for a couple of weeks, and I'm positive their scores would improve straight away.

Ideally, our goal is to turn a weakness into a strength, but it's not always possible. Knowing what you can and can't do is the next best thing. When facing a shot that's not in your wheelhouse, take the conservative approach and wait for another opportunity tailored to a strength. It's called playing smart golf. Zach Johnson knew this and is now a two-time major champion after adding an Open Championship to his resume in 2015 at St Andrews. Not bad for a short-hitting bloke from Iowa.

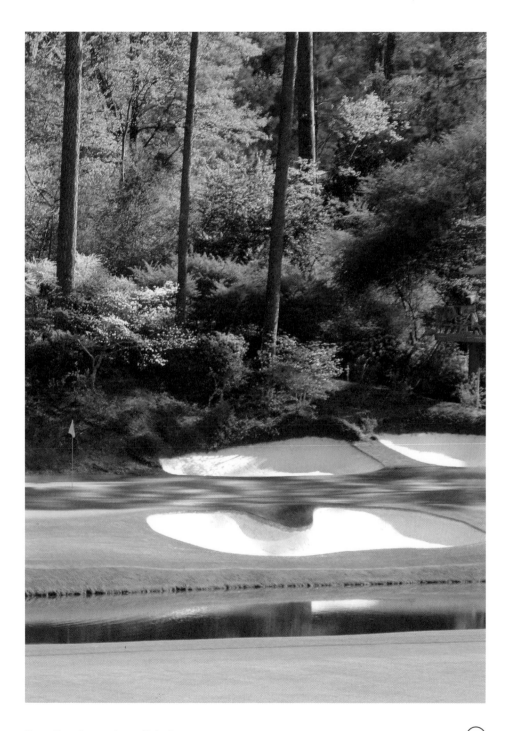

Know Your Strengths and Weaknesses

Par is
Irrelevant –
Sort of

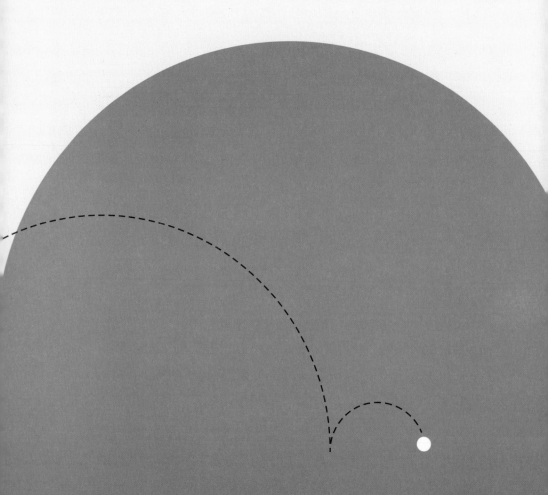

I have a theory about par. It's irrelevant. Attaching a numerical score – par – to a hole implies how it should be played. For instance, a par three should take one shot to reach the green, a par four two shots and a par five three. When really, the goal is to play a hole in the least strokes possible for a player's skill level. If a 550-yard (500-metre) hole was called a par three, would it really matter? It shouldn't, as we'd have to play it the same way as normal, but I'm sure it would freak some people out. As a more realistic example, when a 480-yard (440-metre) hole is called a par four golfers say, 'Geez this is a tough hole', whereas if it's a par five, their thinking changes to, 'This is one of the easier holes on the course.' It all comes down to mindset. As a par four golfers think it'll take two of their finest shots to reach in regulation. As a par five they play it more conservatively, with less stress and usually in fewer strokes.

We can't get rid of par, it's part of the game, the standard for which all scores are based off – but we can rethink it. So, to ease the anxiety on holes you find challenging, play a tough par four as a short par five, or a long par three as a short four. If you receive a stroke based on handicap, why not use it? Often holes with a tougher stroke index have the most double bogies. Partly because, yes, they are more difficult, but also because golfers force the issue by taking too much risk for their ability. Recently I was discussing this with a friend of mine, Mark Rothfield, who's a member at Royal Melbourne. The 2nd hole of the East Course is a par four dogleg to the right, measuring 440 yards (402 metres). The second shot is uphill with a cross bunker that starts about 33 yards (30 metres) short of a very firm green. Mark struggles with this hole and regularly walks off with a 6 or 7 on the scorecard. On handicap, he receives a stroke, so it's very frustrating starting rounds off this way.

Being a par four, he was always tempted to reach it in two shots. This meant cutting the corner of the dogleg with the tee shot, then trying to carry the cross bunker short of the green on the approach. Both shots are dangerous propositions and, even if he managed to navigate them, the green's still extremely difficult to hold with a rescue club or long iron. We spoke about playing it as a three-shot hole or, in other words, a short par five in the following manner. From the tee, take a more conservative line up the left side where there's more room. Then, hit a 7- or 8-iron short of the cross bunker to leave a wedge of some variety for his third. Since adopting this strategy he's regularly scoring 5 net 4, and every so often 4 net 3. It's taken the anxiety out of the hole because he's playing it the way his skill level dictates. Handicaps are there for a reason; sometimes the hardest part is putting the ego aside.

I'd even recommend this strategy for elite amateurs and pros on reachable par fives. My par five scoring average rank on tour was consistently in the top tier even though I was one of the shortest hitters out there. Rather than going for greens in two, I laid up to a good yardage and trusted my wedge game. Par was assured and I regularly made birdie. Sure, eagles were as rare as hen's teeth, but so were bogies and doubles. On tour now, power plays a more important role, but there are still shorter hitters who can compete, although they are becoming fewer and fewer. Brendon Todd's been a great example recently in the US, and my good mate Søren Kjeldsen has been doing it for years on the European Tour. I love watching the women's tours for this reason. They play smarter, with more precision than the men, and are a great example for all golfers to emulate.

The objective is to take big numbers off the card – that's the goal. To write down the lowest score possible, irrelevant of what the par is.

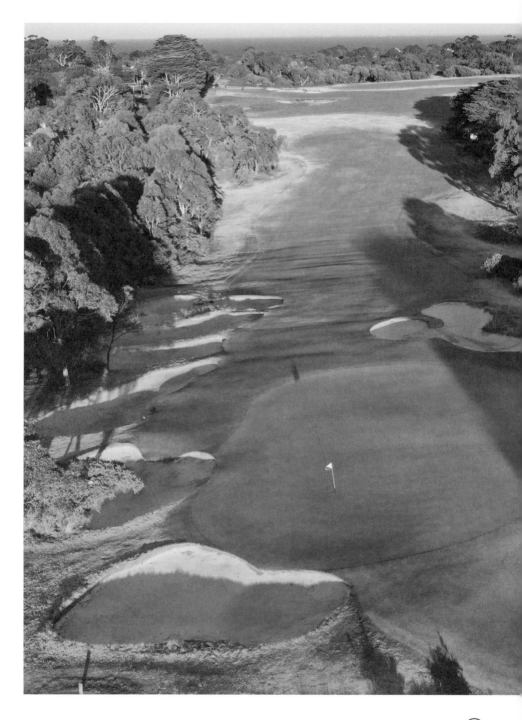

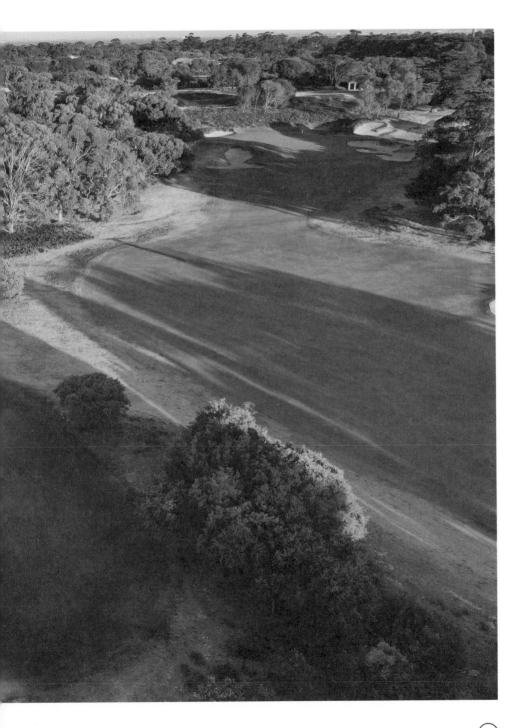

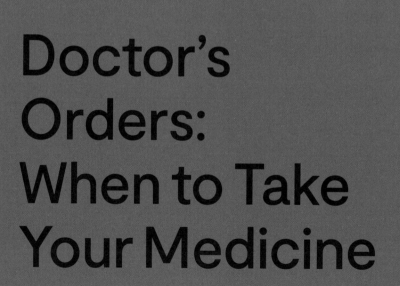

Doctor's Orders: When to Take Your Medicine

As David Toms stood next to his ball on the 72nd hole of the 2001 USPGA Championship, he faced the biggest moment of his career. With a one-shot lead over playing partner Phil Mickelson, all he thought was, 'What's the best way to make four from here?' The 18th hole at the Atlanta Athletic Club that year measured 499 yards (456 metres). As a par four it was a monster hole (an easy par five though as just discussed) and at the time the longest par four in major championship history. After hitting his drive up the right-hand side, David's ball came to rest 234 yards (214 metres) from the hole in the first cut of rough on a slightly downhill lie. The problem – it was all carry since a water hazard protected the front of the green. The lubricated galleries lining the fairway were urging him to go for it, but he knew it was going to come out low bringing in the water, and also the bunkers over the back of the green. Mickelson had a mid-iron left from the middle of the fairway, but David couldn't control what Phil was going to do.

It was fascinating viewing on TV back in my hotel room in Atlanta. As soon as he pulled a wedge from the bag, the commentator began second-guessing him. 'I'm surprised he's laying up,' he said. It took enormous courage to make this decision, and by taking his medicine and backing himself to get the ball up and down from the fairway, worst case he'd be in a playoff.

Mickelson hit a towering 5-iron to the middle of the green 35 feet past the hole. A smart play given the pin was cut only five paces over the water's edge. After laying up short of the water, Toms hit a controlled sand iron from 84 yards (77 metres) finishing 12 feet away. Phil two-putted for par and the stage was set. David calmly stepped up and knocked it in dead centre for his first major title. Afterwards the announcer commended him for the decision to lay up, in spite of his previous comment. It was golf theatre at its finest, and a fitting climax to one of the biggest tournaments in golf.

Perhaps if Jean van de Velde had a similar mindset, things might have worked out differently for him at the Open Championship in 1999 at Carnoustie. All week Jean's French flair was on full display and it was captivating to watch. Standing on the 72nd tee with a 3-shot lead he blocked his drive toward the Barry Burn, a water hazard that snakes its way along the right side of the fairway. Miraculously his ball bounced over the burn and remained dry. After that piece of fortune, you'd think he'd dial things back by playing safely short of the burn, which crossed the fairway 20 yards (18 metres) short of the green, thus taking a big score out of play. Unfortunately, he continued on the only path he knew, hitting 2-iron into the grandstand lining the right side. His ball ricocheted backwards 50 yards (45 metres) short of the green into extremely deep rough, signalling the beginning of the end. His next shot found the burn, and after a penalty drop and two more strokes, he somehow managed to conjure up the fortitude to roll in an 8-footer for a triple bogey 7. Lead gone, playoff forthcoming. Paul Lawrie ended up winning the 4-hole three-man playoff, leaving Jean to reside in the annals of golf's biggest collapses. Like many of the millions of viewers around the world, I was in complete shock. Hindsight's a convenient thing, but I wonder how often his caddy wished after the tee shot he'd given Jean his wedge and putter and said, 'See you on the green!' Golf does crazy things even to the best players.

Payne Stewart faced a similar situation to David Toms in the 1999 US Open at Pinehurst. It even involved the same player, Phil Mickelson. In the final group and with a one-shot lead playing the 72nd hole, Payne found the heavy rough down the right side off the tee on the 446-yard (408-metre) par four. Meanwhile, Phil found the fairway and made a solid par. With no option but to lay up, Payne backed himself to make four the hard way. History shows he wedged his third shot to 15 feet and made a putt so iconic they erected a statue of the pose he struck as the ball went in. Tragically, four months later Payne would lose his life in a freak plane crash. I was fortunate to play with Payne at the 1998 Coolum Classic on the Aussie Tour when he came down for a couple of years to partner his close mate, Todd Woodbridge, in the pro-am format. Payne's swing was as smooth as butter, and his personality meant you couldn't help but love the guy. Later when we moved to the US we lived around the corner from his widow, Tracey, and have been great friends ever since.

I love revisiting key moments in golf history and observing how events unfolded. We can all learn a great deal from the decisions players make in different situations. Knowing when to go for it and when to lay up is *the* conundrum in golf. First, weigh up a shot's risk and reward. Then, assess which has the higher potential for gain or loss.

Drill

Play 9 holes and deliberately miss fairways, and where possible hit into deep rough (strange, I know). From there, play two balls, one aggressively and one conservatively. Tally up both scores at the end of 9 holes and see whether the aggressive or conservative ball wins. Depending on how severe the risk and reward are, I bet the conservative ball wins 80 per cent of the time.

This game gives an insight into when to go for it and when not to. After a while, as you arrive at your ball, you'll get a feel for what the correct play is. Sometimes it just takes exploring both sides of the equation in practice first, to gain the experience for when it arises in competition.

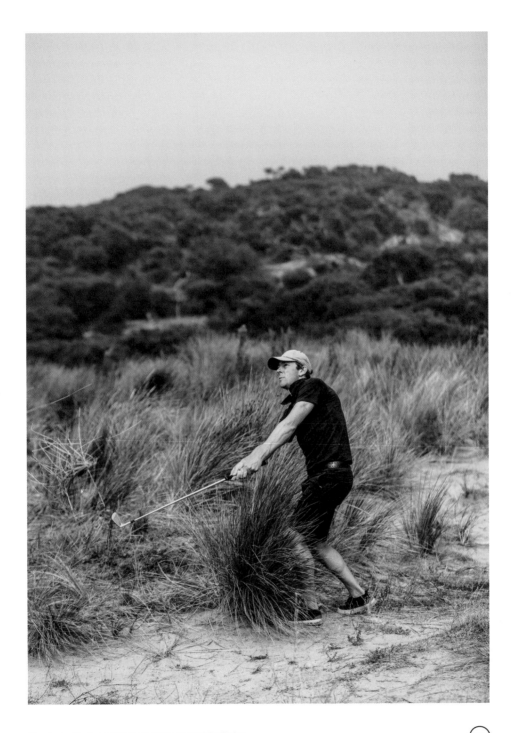

Doctor's Orders: When to Take Your Medicine

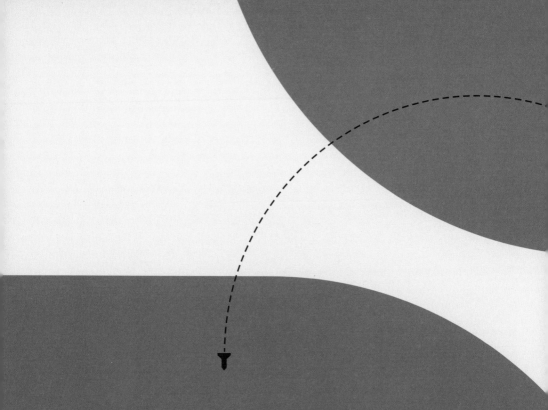

Playing With Your B and C Games

'Golf is not about the quality of your good shots, it's about the quality of your bad ones.' Those words of wisdom from my coach Neil Simpson early on have stuck with me ever since. Let's face it, how often do we have our A game? Not very often, and, trust me, even tour pros rarely fire on all cylinders. When everything's clicking you are in the zone – a state you're lucky to be in a couple of times a year for 9 or 18 holes, let alone for an entire four-day tournament. Forget about it; doesn't happen. The rest of the time we're trying to manage our way around the course as best we can. In my era the golfer who did this better than anyone was Tiger Woods. He's won more than half his tournaments with his B and C games. When his A game did show up, well, it was a case of who's coming second. That's how good Tiger was.

The ability to turn a 74 into 70, or 86 into 80, or 98 into 90, has little to do with technique. It's about the mental side, strategy, the shorter clubs and handling your emotions. Yes, your emotions because golf is a very emotional game. There have been times on the course when I've wanted to snap a club* over my knee or put a hole in the bag with my driver. Come on, you know what I'm talking about. Recognising we're losing it is half the battle because these moments heavily influence our score that day.

Here's an example: Riley's off a 5 handicap, scores in the mid to high 70s on a good day, low 80s on average days, and well into the 80s on bad ones. His full swing is technically sound, but his short game lets him down. Mentally he struggles when things aren't going well from tee to green. And if he doesn't get off to a good start, frustration sets in, thinking it will only get worse. Sound familiar? Here's how to get through these days.

---

*The only time I ever did snap a club (my putter) was after the final round of the Australian Open at Kingston Heath one year. At least I had the sense to snap it after the round rather than during because then I'd have been left putter-less. Mal Purcell, a close friend of mine, heard what I'd done and rummaged it out of the locker room bin. Years later, he presented it to me in its two pieces as a practical joke. All I could think of was how to get rid of it again!

Wedges and in

Firstly, for Riley to turn those 80-plus scores into a few strokes lower, good wedge play and a solid short game are required. Players who score well consistently are handy from wedge distance in. Realistically, Riley's not going to hit the ball well all the time, so on poor ball-striking days the only way to score is with the shorter clubs. For starters, when he does get a chance to practise, structuring his time with this in mind is vital. At least half of this time would be best spent on wedges, chipping, bunker shots and putting (how to divide this time is detailed later in the 'Quality Over Quantity' chapter, page 114).

Every shot counts

Next, and I can't stress this enough, every shot in a round of golf counts. It sounds obvious, but it's often forgotten when things aren't going as planned. During these moments we need to dig deep and have a 'never give up' attitude because strokes can easily be given away. Players think, 'I just don't have it today', and aren't fully committed or, worse, give up. The beauty of golf is that you never know when one swing or shot can turn things around. All of a sudden you hit a pure 5-iron and go, 'Aha, there's the feeling I'm after!' But whoops, you just bogeyed the last 4 holes straight after playing carelessly. It's why a full commitment to every shot is critical. The 'feel' can come at any moment. If you shoot 78 for the day, do you think the 53rd shot is more or less important than the 21st one? Of course not. Every shot matters. Developing a mindset and routine for consistently committing to each shot is an important key to scoring.

This comes back to pre-shot routines (PSRs) and the acceptance aspect I spoke of in *Tour Mentality*. In a nutshell, the 30- to 60-second period around every shot is all you can control – especially accepting the result. How you react to results has a huge influence in toning down the negative emotional elements to the game, such as anger, frustration and pessimism. Accepting the result, good or bad, smooths the way for a better attitude – and better score.

'Pars never hurt
us and sometimes
bogies are just fine.
It's the double bogies
and worse that
ruin scorecards.'

Strategy

The final piece when we don't have our A game is strategy. Players who score well figure out quickly what's working and what isn't, and adapt accordingly. For example, if the driver's uncooperative, let's put a 3-wood or hybrid in to play off the tee instead. Sure, we'll be further back for the approach but at least in the fairway where it's easier to score from than the trees. Also, learn how to hit what I call a 'fairway finder'. For me this was a low fade I could consistently put in play, almost like a punch shot but with a driver. It takes a little practice on the range to figure out, but well worth it when you can't find the planet with the big stick. When our irons are off, playing toward the safer side of a green is smart. On sandbelt courses here in Melbourne, for example, 40 feet below the hole is much better than 10 feet above it. Even missing a green on the correct side is a better play. If you're hitting the ball well, then be more aggressive, but if you haven't hit a solid iron shot all day, a more conservative approach is best. Pars never hurt us and sometimes bogies are just fine. It's the double bogies and worse that ruin scorecards. If you short-side yourself, and don't have the perfect lie, stay away from the hero shot. Instead, choose the higher percentage chip or bunker shot and play for 15–20 feet past the pin. It takes the big number out of play, and more often than not, you knock it closer anyway.

Some of my most satisfying rounds were one or 2 under par when I simply had no right to sign for anything below 75. These came about through managing my game based on what I had on the day. Then, hopefully by the following morning, everything was right with the world (and my game) again.

Rain, Hail
or Shine

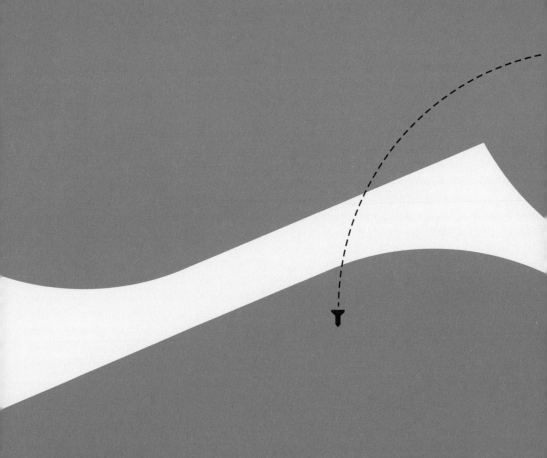

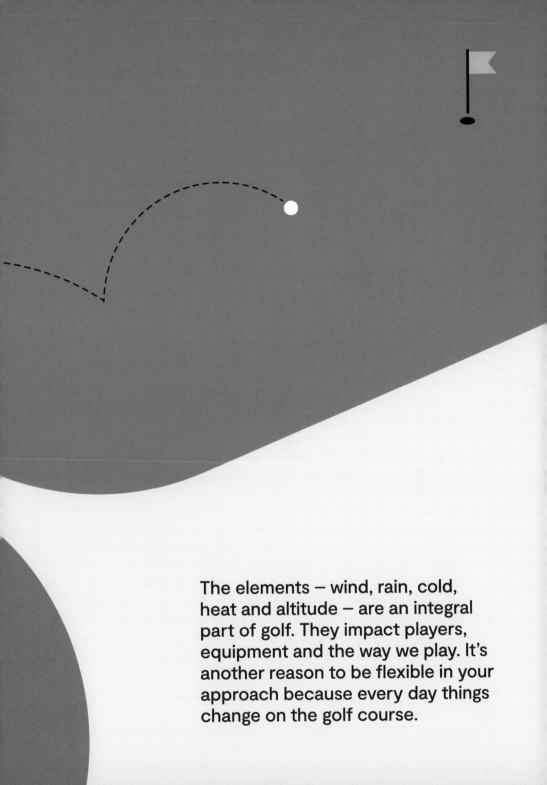

The elements – wind, rain, cold, heat and altitude – are an integral part of golf. They impact players, equipment and the way we play. It's another reason to be flexible in your approach because every day things change on the golf course.

Wind

Knowing how to control your ball in the wind is essential to scoring. In an earlier chapter I spoke about using the wind to your advantage from off the tee and into the green (page 23 and 26). With driver on downwind tee shots, tee it higher, move the ball position an inch forward, and drop the right shoulder a touch for a higher launch angle. Hitting up on the ball promotes the higher flight and downwind; the longer the ball stays in the air the better. For irons it's simply taking a club or two less (higher in loft) to allow for the extra carry. The good news when playing downwind is miss-hit shots curving offline are straightened up.

When playing into the wind, miss-hits are exaggerated. A solid strike and controlling spin are paramount, otherwise things can get ugly. For driver into the wind, tee it lower, shift the ball position back an inch and focus on good rhythm. For irons, the solution is a three-quarter knockdown shot. For example, if you have 7-iron into a green with some wind in your face, take a 5- or 6-iron, narrow your stance a little (for more control) and focus on a smooth three-quarter swing. There's a reason for the saying 'Swing it easy when it's breezy'. By reducing clubhead speed, less spin is imparted on the ball and the wind doesn't affect it as much. It flies lower and releases more, so factor this in too.

Golfers think the knockdown shot is more for elite players, but believe me, anyone can learn it and, when the wind's really pumping, it's an invaluable shot. I played in the 2019 Victorian PGA with a good mate of mine, Jonathan 'Rosho' Rosham, at the Cape Schanck Golf Club on the Mornington Peninsula an hour south-east of Melbourne. It's a pro-am format like the Dunhill Links on the European Tour, and during the third round winds gusting up to 70 km/h brought many of the pros to their knees. Rosho was off a 15 handicap at the time, and we'd been working on his knockdown shot leading up to the tournament knowing we could get a day such as this. On the par-three 13th hole all that hard work was rewarded. From an elevated tee, the hole is totally exposed to the elements and requires supreme control of your ball flight. Our two pro playing partners were losing balls way left and right, then Rosho got up and hit a knockdown 7-iron 120 yards (110 metres) under the wind to 10 feet. It was one of the prettiest shots I've seen in such horrific conditions.

The natural tendency is to force shots into the wind by hitting them harder, but this imparts more spin on the ball, bringing the wind into play even more. So, our main focus into the wind is rhythm and tempo. In very strong winds, it can mean using two, three or even four clubs more than usual. The 'Five clubs to one target' drill I had Richie Fulmer do (page 58) is ideal practice for this. Hitting a 5-iron to a 120-metre target on a calm day (when you normally hit it 175 yards (160 metres) requires the rhythm and tempo we're looking for. Who are the best wind players? Look no further than multiple winners of the Open Championship – Peter Thomson, Jack Nicklaus, Tom Watson, Nick Faldo and Tiger Woods from the past 70 years or so answer that question.

Rain

In the US I rarely played in the rain. The PGA Tour's schedule follows the warmer weather, and rain usually meant a thunderstorm, which usually meant play suspended. In Europe and here in Australia, it's rare to have a thunderstorm halt play. Typically, it's just rain, so we keep playing. When conditions are wet the ball doesn't travel as far, for a couple of reasons, so club selection becomes important. Moisture fills the grooves on the clubface creating a deadening effect, while extra layers of clothing can restrict your swing's range of motion. Also, be aware with the driver – a wet clubface can squirt the ball off in unusual directions, so make sure to keep it dry before hitting. I've seen plenty of players taking a couple of practice swings in the rain, and by the time they address the ball, the clubface has streaks of moisture all over it, resulting in very ordinary shots from good swings.

For shots into and around greens there's the skid factor. Since the ball can't penetrate and grip the wet surface, it skids, scooting it on further. You must allow for this. Likewise, morning dew has a similar affect.

Mud balls are another factor in wet conditions. There's no exact science to them, but I go by the 'mud right/ ball left' theory. Meaning, if mud's clumped on the right-hand side of the ball, it will veer left. How much depends on the amount of mud and the position on the ball. It's a best-guess scenario, but it definitely affects a ball's flight. The worst mud balls I ever encountered were at TPC Sawgrass during The Players Championship some years ago before course renovations made playing conditions firmer. It poured down and given the PGA Tour likes to think of its event as the fifth major, preferred lies were not allowed. Seeing balls nose- dive into water hazards from good shots wasn't much fun, let me tell you. If you get a mud ball in practice, don't wipe it off. Hit the shot and see what happens. It might provide some insight for one in competition.

Cold

As with rain, club selection is all important in cold weather because the ball doesn't go as far for the following reasons:

1. Energy transfer between club and ball is not as efficient.

2. Cold air is more dense than warm air, creating extra friction and drag on the ball.

3. Your muscles are tighter, resulting in a shorter swing with less speed.

How much distance is lost due to these factors depends on the temperature and your swing speed. For scientific golfers out there, the Titleist website offers facts and figures on all this. As a feel player, after a couple of holes I have a good sense how far the ball is travelling on chilly days. Either way, the ability to make adjustments on the fly is all part of knowing your own game. Before governing bodies changed the rules, heat sachets were permitted in pockets as a way to keep your hands warm. Caddies would even put balls in with them to heat them up. Unfortunately, the sachets are now seen as an aid and have been banned in pro golf, but they may still be allowed at amateur level. Typically, the coldest tournament is the European Tour's Dunhill Links Championship in Scotland held during October each year. The combination of cold, wind and rain makes for a very trying week. However, playing these historic courses softens the blow – and a wee dram of whisky in the evenings doesn't hurt either. ☺

Heat

For the same reasons the ball flies less in cold weather, the opposite is true in warmer conditions:

1. The ball comes off with extra velocity and spin because energy transfer is more efficient.

2. There's less friction in the air.

3. Our bodies are more flexible and responsive.

How much again depends on how hot it is and swing speed. Humidity has an effect too, but it's very minimal. In humid conditions the ball flies further because water weighs less than the nitrogen and oxygen molecules in dry air, meaning that when it's humid you're hitting into thinner air. The difference is barely noticeable though, only one yard or so from no humidity to full humidity. If you're good enough to factor that in, then I tip my hat to you. The toughest part about humid conditions is keeping your hands and grips dry from sweat. It's a good idea to carry extra gloves in the bag, since they become drenched easily. If you've played in parts of Queensland, Asia and Florida, you know what I mean.

Altitude

Altitude, along with wind, has the greatest influence on the distance a ball travels. As a general rule, for every 1000 feet (or about 300 metres) above sea level, the ball flies two per cent further. For example, the European Tour's event at Crans-sur-Sierre in Switzerland is played at roughly 5000 feet (1525 metres) above sea level. This equates to the ball flying about 10 per cent further, a necessary consideration for club selection. If your 7-iron flies 164 yards (150 metres), then it's 180 yards (165 metres) at this altitude. That's a huge difference. Uphill shots aren't affected as much because the ball's not in the air as long, while downhill ones – well, it feels like they may never land. Crans-sur-Sierre is an amazing town, with what feels like some of the cleanest air I've ever breathed. If you happen to visit, take the cable car up the mountain to the glacier for astonishing views. The course is fun to play – the surrounding alps make an idyllic setting, and it's always nice to see your driving distance stats go up at week's end.

Golf is fascinating in how it throws up different conditions and situations to deal with each time we play. The ability to interpret, adapt to and solve each unique challenge is integral to playing and scoring well.

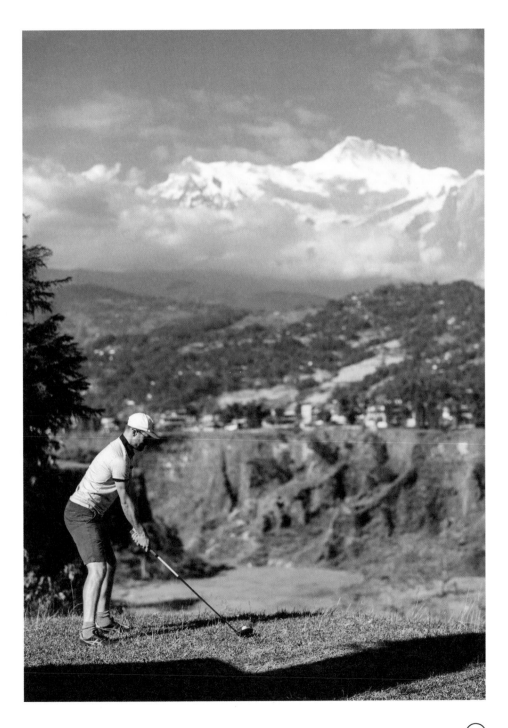

Rain, Hail or Shine

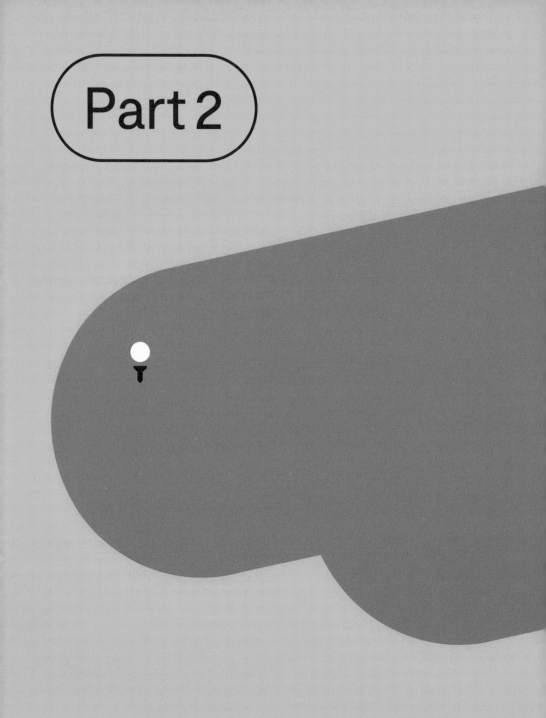

Part 2

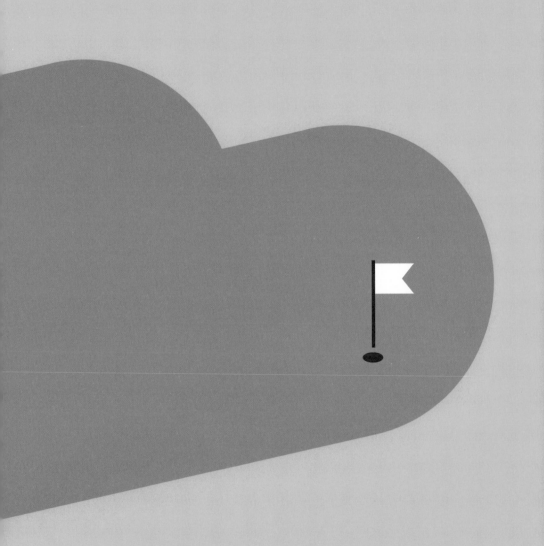

Preparation

Warming Up

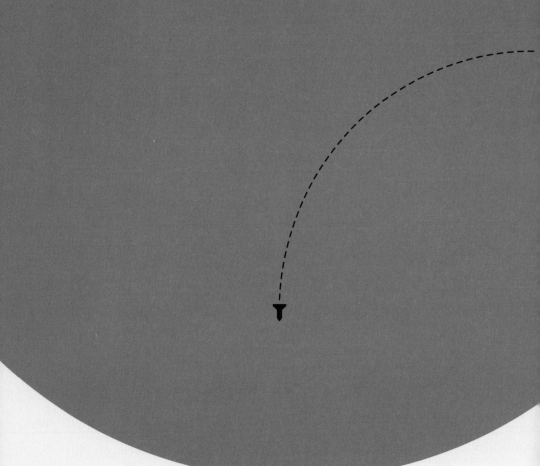

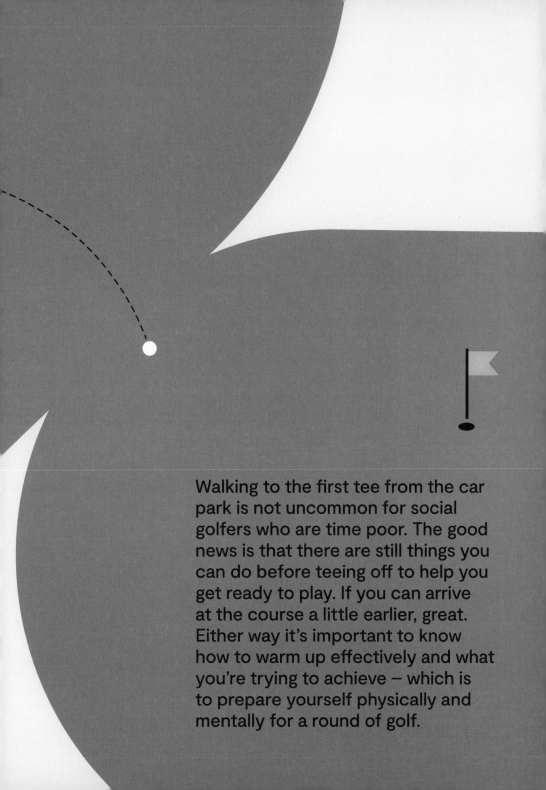

Walking to the first tee from the car park is not uncommon for social golfers who are time poor. The good news is that there are still things you can do before teeing off to help you get ready to play. If you can arrive at the course a little earlier, great. Either way it's important to know how to warm up effectively and what you're trying to achieve — which is to prepare yourself physically and mentally for a round of golf.

Firstly, do some form of stretching prior to playing. How much depends on time, but even a couple of basic golf stretches in the locker room or beside the first tee can help prevent injury when you decide to lash away at one on the opening hole. Ideally, do some light aerobic exercise first because stretching cold muscles can lead to straining areas that aren't yet warm and pliable. Something that gets the blood flowing to the various muscle tissue is ideal, such as walking or riding a stationary bike for five minutes. Jumping jacks or high knees (jogging on the spot) for a minute or so has a similar effect, and for those with bad knees (like me), air squats do the job.

Once warm, we can now stretch effectively, and I recommend dynamic stretching before a round. If you've seen Miguel Ángel Jiménez's stretching routine on the range, you'll see him doing a variety of unique dynamic stretches (typically with a cigar in his mouth). Static stretching involves holding the stretch for an extended period. Save these for afterwards because studies have shown they can reduce power if done beforehand. Dynamic stretches are controlled movements to promote range of motion. Start slow and ease your way into them. Experiment with different stretches to find out which best suit you and try to be consistent with them before playing.

Some of the best for golf are:

- **Lunge with a twist**: Hold each end of a club horizontally out in front of you. Step your right leg forward into a lunge and rotate your upper body to the right. Repeat with the left leg.
- **Side bends**: Hold each end of a club horizontally above your head and slowly lean left and then right stretching from side to side.
- **Swing two clubs together**: Take two wedges and slowly start swinging them, letting the weight pull your body through the range of motion (at the very least do this if you have no time before teeing off). Don't stop the motion, make it continual so you are swinging right- and left-handed back and through.
- **Elastic resistance bands**: These are great for activating your golf muscles and there are various exercises you can do with them. Check out the MyTPI website for plenty of golf-related ones.

After stretching I've created three different warm-ups of five, 15 and 45 minutes, based on the amount of time I have prior to teeing off. The 45-minute version is what I used throughout my playing career, and for avid golfers, high-level amateurs and pros, it's a useful template to work off. Some players take longer, some shorter. Again, find what works for you, but for me this amount of time is ideal. It commences when I arrive at the range and ends as I step on to the first tee.

45-MINUTE WARM-UP

To begin, I hit balls on the range for 20 minutes starting with a 54-degree wedge. A wedge is great for getting the golf muscles going and it's easy to find the clubface with it. Then, I work down through the bag going to a 7-iron, 3-iron, driver, back to a 6-iron, and finishing with the club I have for the first shot of the day, typically driver. All up, I hit about 35 balls. Going through the different clubs provides a good cross-section of the various ones I'll use throughout the round. With each club I have a target to aim at, but I'm not too concerned with being precise until I start hitting 6-irons toward the end. With these I go through my full pre-shot routine (PSR) for five balls to get in game mode. My final swing replicates the first shot of the day – this way I'm ready for what lies ahead on the first tee. If it's a par four or five, I visualise the fairway between two targets on the range. A par three, then I'll picture the green. Throughout, I'm not fazed if the ball isn't going where it's supposed to. This is one of the toughest things for golfers to come to grips with, but I've had great rounds after awful warm-ups and poor rounds after flushing it, so I'm not too fussed if I'm not hitting the ball well. Our goal is to get a feel for the clubface, prime the mind and body, and be in game mode by the end of the warm-up.

From there it's over to the short game area for 10 minutes of chipping and bunker shots to get a feel for the grass, sand and how the ball's reacting. The last 15 minutes is spent on the putting green, rolling putts of varying lengths to gauge the speed of the greens. During the last few minutes, I switch to one ball, and putt to a number of different holes going through my full PSR again to get in game mode. Then, it's off to the first tee.

That's my tournament warm-up. It works for me; it may not for you, but it's something to ponder and tinker with. Some pros only need 30 minutes to warm up, others two hours and everything in between. Tiger Woods's warm-up, for example, is a little under an hour and he reverses this order by starting on the putting green doing some feel and technical work. Then, he moves to the short-game area for chipping and bunker shots. Next, it's on to the range starting with a 56-degree wedge, then 8-iron, 4-iron, 5-wood, 3-wood, driver, back to 8-iron, 56-degree wedge, and finally the driver to replicate his first tee shot. He likes to hit a variety of shapes and trajectories: high, low, draw, fade and combinations of each. Then, he returns to the putting green to roll a few more of varying lengths, and heads to the first tee.

Currently, I notice many pros using a TrackMan device to get their distances dialled in for the day. If that helps them, great. I lean more toward the old-school style warm-up. Peter Thomson used to say all he focused on was a nice light grip pressure and getting loose. Whatever your preference, having a routine is important. It provides a level of comfort – finding one that works for you just takes a little experimentation. Try longer and shorter warm-ups to see which benefits you the most. Now that I play more social golf, I find a 15-minute warm-up is plenty to get ready for a game.

15-MINUTE WARM-UP

Take a 7-iron and driver to the range and do a scaled-down version of the 45-minute warm-up. Fifteen to 20 balls are enough to get the muscles warm and body loose. Start by chipping a few 7-irons and work your way up into full swings before finishing off with some drivers. It's the club we use most often for full swings throughout the round. The goal is to find a nice rhythm and tempo — don't worry about where the ball's going. For the last few minutes roll a few putts of differing lengths to gauge the speed of the greens.

FIVE-MINUTE WARM-UP

This one is simply to get the body moving. If there's a net nearby, hit about a dozen 7-irons in there, focusing on rhythm and tempo. Leave the driver in the bag. When I need to warm up quickly a fun drill is placing three to five balls in a diagonal line away from me, each ball spaced about 6 inches to a foot apart. With a 7-iron hit each ball without stopping the swing. It's like a golf dance where I take my time and step toward the next ball after hitting the previous one. I repeat this a couple of times to elevate the heart rate while also creating clubface awareness. If there's no net and the range is a fair distance away, just roll some putts instead, focusing on speed, rhythm and tempo. On the first hole, ease your way into the round with a club you feel comfortable with. It might be a 5-iron, fairway wood or driver. Focus on a smooth swing, don't try and crush it. Wait until you've hit a few shots on the course before upping the ante.

Depending on your skill level and how warm you feel, navigate the opening hole(s) accordingly. Being aggressive early on probably isn't the wisest approach if you're not warmed up properly or feeling uncomfortable. If the first hole is a par four and your handicap allows a stroke, play it conservatively, even as a par five, for a net par four. Net pars won't hurt you. Starting with a couple of wipes or double bogeys, however, can set the tone for the round, even though it shouldn't. I find good scores develop after a steady start. Rarely do we get off to a hot start and keep it going, especially if we're not fully warmed up. By working your way into the round, it gives you the best chance of having a good day.

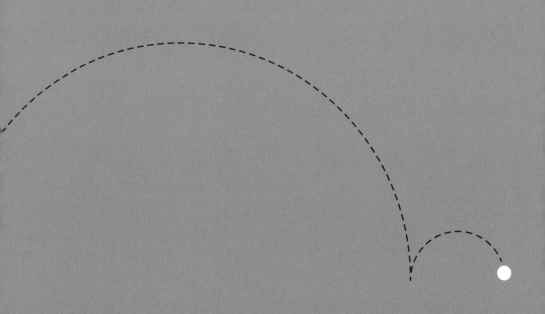

Prepare
for Success

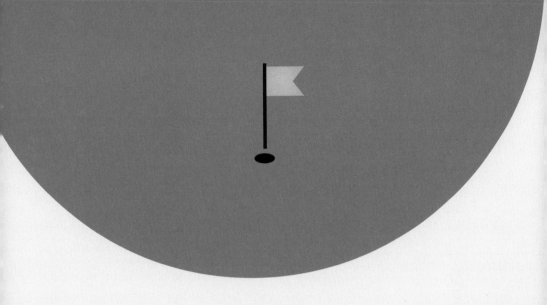

There's an old saying: 'Never hit a shot on the course you haven't hit in practice.' It's great advice, even though almost impossible to do because scenarios arise every now and then that would take an incredibly creative imagination to think of prior. However, being as prepared as possible makes them less stressful when they do appear. This also involves how you prepare in the weeks leading up to an important event or round. It might be your club championship, state title, national open or a major championship. No matter the event, a number of things can be done beforehand to help you perform well.

In the weeks leading up to certain events, I'd map out strategies for areas of my game needing extra attention. For example, being in the fairway at US Opens is essential, so I'd find (or visualise) the narrowest fairways to hit down with driver and 3-wood. A great course for this was near where I lived in Orlando, Florida, called Orange Tree. Payne Stewart used to play there in preparation for his US Opens – after playing there a few times I understood why. If you hit driver off every tee and avoid a penalty stroke for 18 holes, you're good to go! Payne's two US Open titles certainly are testament to this.

Harbour Town Golf Links at Hilton Head has very small greens tough to hit in regulation, so more short-game work was appropriate knowing I'd have plenty of up and downs to navigate during the tournament. On courses with huge putting surfaces, extra time on long lag putting is necessary. The Old Course at St Andrews is a prime example with 7 double greens* of enormous size. I even carried two putters there during the Dunhill Links Championship a couple of times because 80-footers (and longer) were quite common and swinging my broomstick putter far enough back on the slower greens was a struggle. I took out my 4-iron and put a regular length putter in the bag to counteract this. It didn't matter which iron I dropped because the Old Course requires plenty of imagination and rarely calls for normal stock shots.

---

*An interesting fact at the Old Course is all the double greens combine hole numbers that add up to 18. The 2nd and 16th holes are a double green, the 3rd and 15th, 4th and 14th, 5th and 13th, 6th and 12th, 7th and 11th, and the 8th and 10th holes. Not sure if it was done on purpose or it just worked out that way, but it's a fascinating tidbit. For more such insights into the Old Course, *The Spirit of St Andrews* by Alister MacKenzie is a book well worth reading.

At Augusta National the severely sloping lies are a major challenge (TV doesn't do the course justice in this regard). Leading up to The Masters I'd look for slopes to hit off any chance I got. That and rolling putts on a concrete floor to get a feel for how quick the greens would be. On renowned windy venues extra work on low knockdown shots in the lead-up was part of a practice session. I never enjoyed playing in wet-weather gear but it is part of the game, so rainy practice days were perfect preparation. In a nutshell, when you tick as many boxes as possible, knowing the work's been done is a powerful asset in competition.

During tournament week, preparation centred around fine-tuning my game for scoring. I didn't do a lot of practice on the Tuesday and Wednesday before a tournament; that was for off weeks. The focus was on playing holes to adjust to course conditions, short game and just hitting enough balls on the range to keep my swing in check. I heard stories about how players would rarely see Jack Nicklaus on the range during tournaments, and same goes for Annika Sörenstam. They worked extremely hard on their games away from tournament weeks, while during events they wanted to be fresh for the four days ahead.

The night before a round I looked at what I ate and how much exercise I did to see what worked best. I found watching a movie (if I was on the road) always helped take my mind away from golf – it doesn't help to be constantly thinking about it. The day of a tournament round was much of the same. For a morning tee time, waking up three hours beforehand allowed my body time to get going, so I never felt rushed before getting to the course. That meant for a 7 am tee time, a 4 am alarm was set, so getting to bed early the night before was taken into account. An afternoon tee time gave me a chance to meditate in the morning. I discovered meditation early in my career on the European Tour and, after doing an introductory course with Eric Harrison at the Perth Meditation Centre, kept at it from there. Through meditation the stressful moments on course weren't such a big deal. It provided an awareness to my thoughts and overall calmness that paid dividends as my career progressed.

Getting back to game day, once at the course, I had a set amount of time to do all my pre-game work. Stretching, eating, applying sunscreen and so on, before heading to the practice area to start the warm-up. This entire process was developed so by the time I stepped onto the first tee I was ready for a good day of golf. Preparation is a vital ingredient to becoming a complete player. This is what worked for me, and again, your goal is to find what works for you.

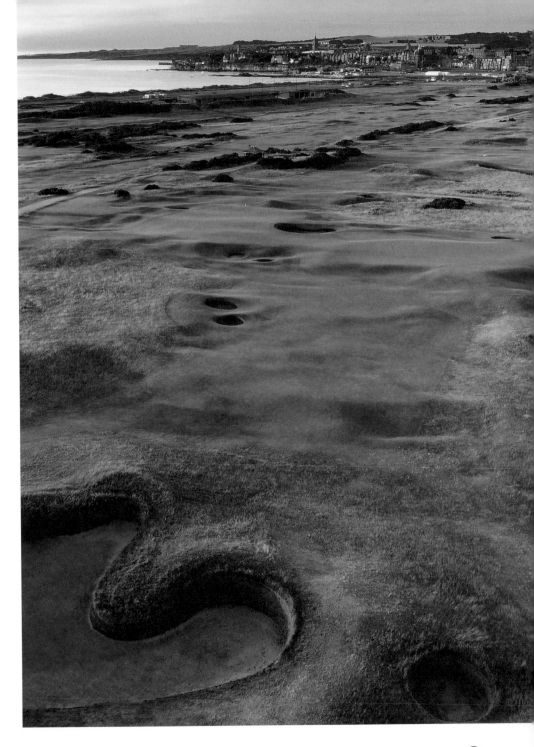

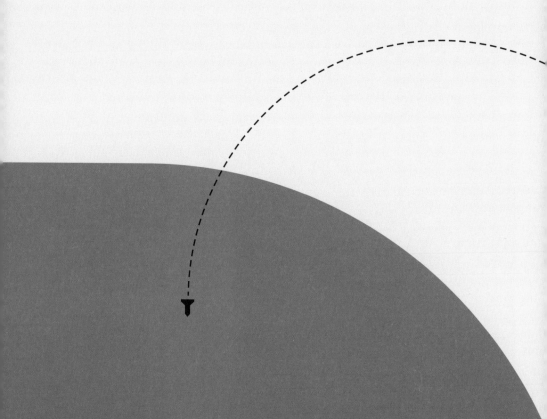

Get Better
Every Day

I love listening to podcasts and discussions in general about developing the mind, body and spirit. TED Talks are a great platform for all this and, a few years ago, I came across an intriguing one by former pro tennis player Eric Butorac. His name may not ring too many bells unless you follow tennis closely, but his journey to excellence is absorbing. Eric played for a Division 3 College and, in his own words, 'Division 3 tennis players don't go pro.' His talk focused on winning the daily battles. People always dream big and look years ahead to goals they want to achieve. But are they achievable right now? Probably not. By setting daily attainable goals, it enables us to 'win each day'. This way we're not failing all the time (if for example the goal is to be No. 1 in the world). Instead, we're accomplishing something every single day, creating a powerful mindset to continue building upon. Check out Eric's talk. It's a unique take on being successful in sport from someone more like the vast majority of the population than the naturally gifted select few.

Similar to Eric, throughout my playing career I had a simple philosophy: how can I get better today? When I went to bed at night, my goal was to be better than when I woke up that morning. Structuring each day with this in mind was the catalyst for gradual improvement throughout my career. I never climbed three or four rungs of the ladder at once, only one at a time, and for extended periods I'd be on that rung for a while before moving up to the next one. Progress was slow but steady, and the foundation for my consistency over many years.

Sometimes the improvements were so small it seemed there weren't any advances being made. But I knew better because progress doesn't always have to be physical, tangible things such as changes in technique. Some days my goal was simply to stay in the present as often as possible, or remember to take a deep, relaxing breath at the start of my PSR. Other times it would be to learn a new skill, like how to play greenside bunker shots with a 3-iron, or to do an extra set of reps at the gym. At the end of each day I'd review everything and was able to feel a sense of accomplishment. I'd set a goal, achieved it and knew I'd won the day. This built confidence, and by continually adding these days up over time, I improved.

A critical element to delivering on this strategy is having a plan. In the morning write it out; then in the evening, review how things went. What worked, what didn't and areas needing further attention. Change things up regularly too. With gym exercise for example, stimulating different muscles promotes growth and progression. With golf it's the same, by working on different areas of the game and thinking outside the box.

Did I set long-term goals? Yes, but then I broke them down into more immediate, achievable goals that could be completed today, then the next day and so on. By focusing on what we can control (that is, the present moment), the long-term goal simply takes care of itself. This approach applies exactly the same way to the PSR. Control the process in the present moment and the result takes care of itself. Add these quality PSRs up at the end of 18 holes, and our score is the result.

In any case, if you start each day by saying 'How can I better today?', you can't go wrong. Progress is inevitable; trust me, I know.

'A critical element to delivering on this strategy is having a plan. In the morning write it out; then in the evening, review how things went – what worked, what didn't and areas needing further attention.'

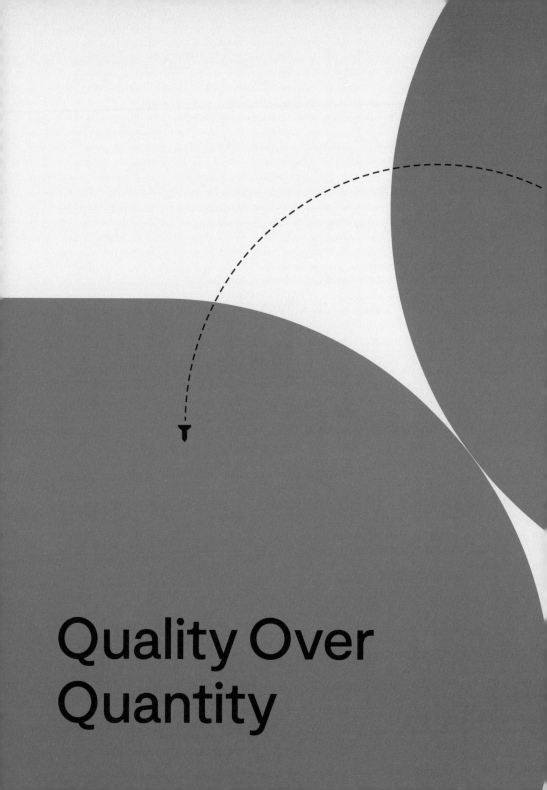

Quality Over
Quantity

Following on from the last chapter, getting the most out of a practice session is our goal. But how do we do that? Firstly, as mentioned, a clear plan is recommended. Writing it out beforehand and checking off each area along the way helps provide a sense of accomplishment as the session progresses. It's also a reference to fall back on when we start going off on a tangent. For example, we may start off saying, 'For these 10 balls I'm going to work on my takeaway.' After four shots, the ball is not going where it's supposed to, so we wonder why and start experimenting. 'I'll just hit a few balls trying this,' and 20 balls later we're tied in knots. I've been here – this is the main reason for writing out a plan beforehand. When you inevitably veer off track it helps to get back to the original agenda.

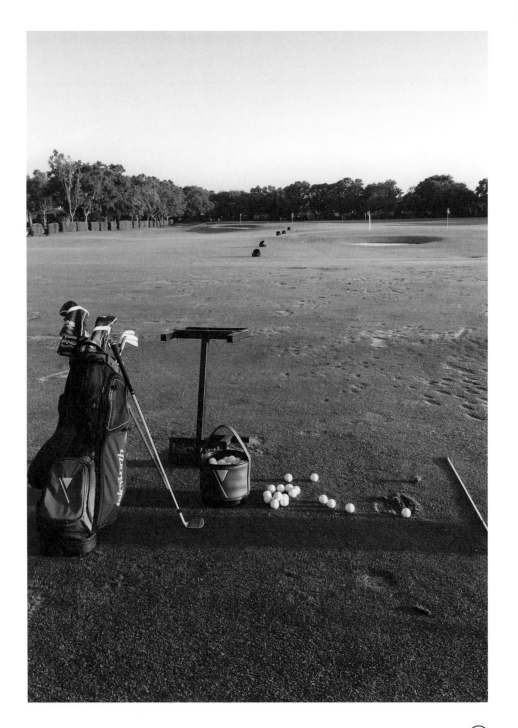

Secondly, the plan needs a productive structure covering areas that stimulate improvement. The majority of golfers work only on technique. Yes, technique is important, but it can be all-consuming and easy to go off on the aforementioned tangents. Allocate time in the session for skill and competitive work. They're essential to becoming a complete golfer on the course. You wouldn't believe how many times someone's said to me, 'I hit the ball great on the range, but can't do it on the course.' In other words, they are driving-range golfers. They make it look easy on the range but can't shoot a decent score on the course. Our goal is the opposite. Be okay with looking ordinary on the range with the purpose of playing well and shooting good scores on the course. To achieve this, structure practice by dividing time into the following three key areas – technique, skills and competition.

I understand having a practice structure isn't for everyone. For some people it drives them crazy, but for others it's essential. Once again, the key is to figure out what works for you. Here is an example of the structure I use to work on full swing for an hour. Use it as a template to build your own if you like the sound of it.

TECHNIQUE

For the first 20 minutes focus on technique, as it lays the foundation for the remainder of the session. The hardest part is not caring where the ball goes during this time. Hitting into a net is ideal because it allows you to focus solely on the physical moves/feels being worked on. Also, exaggerate these moves/feels. Making changes in technique takes time and the quickest way to implement them is by overdoing things. Feel and reality are two different things. I've videoed golfers and asked them to exaggerate what they feel. In reality they come nowhere close. By overdoing it, when going back to your normal swing the moves/feels are closer to working their way in. Over an extended period, you may go too far, so just keep a check on this from time to time with your coach or on video.

SKILLS

After technique , focus on skill work for the next 20 minutes. This time is for creativity, to have fun and experiment with different shots.

The 'one club to five targets' drill (opposite page) teaches clubface awareness, and how to execute different shots that are very useful for the course. For example, when you're in the trees and need to punch out through a gap, a low half-swing 6-iron is the shot. But how often do you practise this? Never, I'm guessing. Other shots rarely worked on are from sloping lies, fairway bunkers, out of the rough and the like. The same goes for short game. There's a variety of skill drills to try. The idea is to be as creative as possible and have fun.

Drill

One club to five targets: The reverse of the 'Five clubs to one target' drill I mentioned on page 29. For example, with 6-iron, hit five balls to a target 55 yards (50 metres) away, then five balls to a target at 87 yards (80 metres), then to targets at 120 yards (110 metres), 153 yards (140 metres) and 186 yards (170 metres). With each target try different trajectories and shapes – high draws, low fades and so on. For fun, see if you can hit a full 6-iron 55 yards (50 metres). How do you do that? Open the face way up, aim miles left and swing away. You may shank or duff a few, but soon you'll hit one just right and hey presto – it's a 55-yard flop shot with a 6-iron! I love making practice as hard as possible so when I'm on the course, things seem easier. Plus, if you can hit a 6-iron flop shot consistently, just imagine how simple a regular flop shot with a sand wedge will become.

COMPETITION

The last 20 minutes is for competitive work. Here we hit shots that require a result to create some pressure. On the range it's easy to hit the ball well and get in a groove if there's nothing riding on it. On the course, however, there's always a result involved, so practising with something on the line helps us become more accustomed to it. Working on PSRs here is crucial too because we rely on these when nervous or uncomfortable about a shot on the course. My favourite competitive drill for full shots is the 'Three-in-a-row' drill (see opposite page).

Technique, skills and competition: three areas to work on during every session for each part of your game – full swing, chipping, bunkers, wedges and putting. Ideally, divide your time for each into thirds. However, be flexible depending on where your game is at. For example, when working on technical changes, I'd recommend a 30-minute: 15-minute: 15-minute ratio for technique, skills and competition (even 40:10:10). If you're fine-tuning for a competition, then a 15:15:30 ratio is ideal to spend more time on the competitive element.

In summary, exaggerate technique, get creative with skill work and put yourself under some pressure with competitive games. If you follow this structure, I guarantee you will be better at the end of every session than at the start.

Drill

Three in a row: Choose two targets in the distance to hit three shots in a row between. Vary the width of the targets depending on the club and shot being attempted. Don't make it too easy, or impossible either. For example, I wouldn't pick a 10-metre-wide gap to hit three high-draw drivers between, as you could be there all day. Conversely, don't give yourself the width of the 1st fairway at St Andrews. You could do that with your eyes closed. The goal is to make it difficult enough to feel uncomfortable on the third and final attempt. Miss, and start again. Sounds simple, but it can get frustrating after missing the third attempt a few times. These are the same emotions we feel on the course. Focus on the process (your PSR) and let the result take care of itself. After completing the drill, next time that shot comes up in competition, you'll feel confident knowing you've already done it in practice.

Part 3

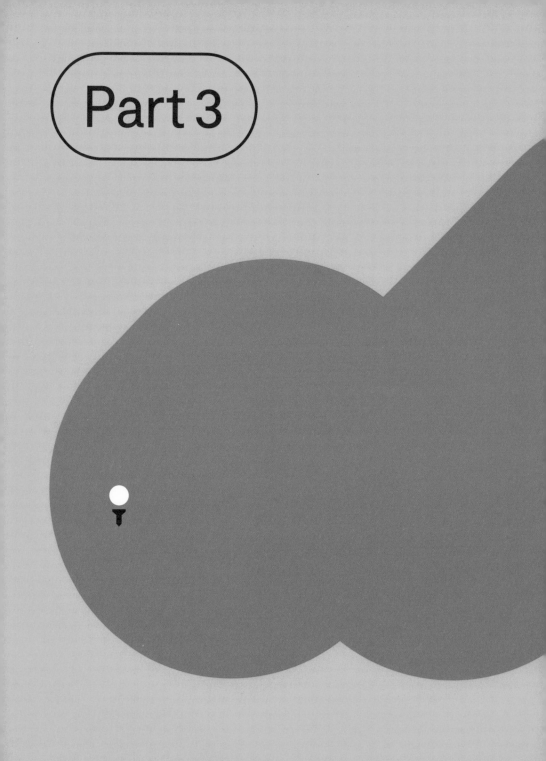

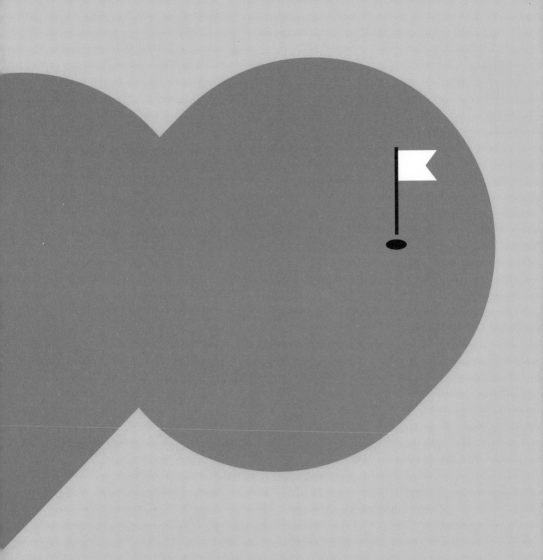

Mental

Striving for
Perfection

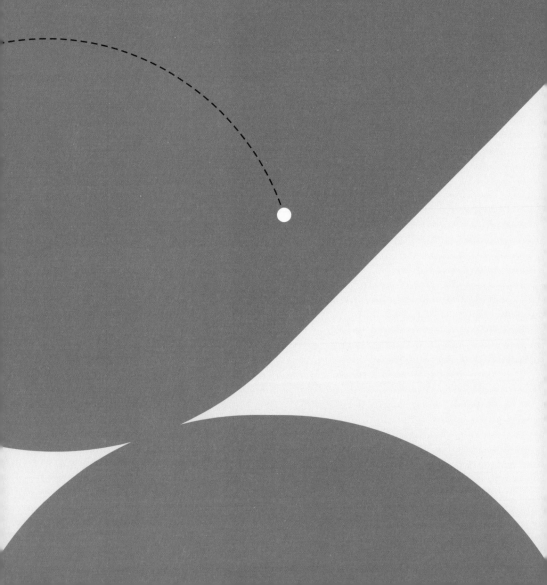

Herb Elliott, one of Australia's greatest middle-distance runners, wrote the introduction for *Winning Attitudes*, a book on performance and achievement in sport. The information within is timeless and from a variety of proven sources. Herb's introduction includes a reflection on fellow Aussie legend and swimming great Shane Gould. He'd always been curious as to what drove Shane's mental process and how she was able to achieve three gold medals, a silver and a bronze at the 1972 Olympic Games in Munich all at the age of 15.

Initially, Herb wasn't having much luck getting Shane to explain her approach until she said, 'Of course, whenever I went into the pool to train, I aimed for perfection with every stroke.' In that moment he discovered what separated her from the rest. She was striving to be perfect with every single stroke in the pool. 'Practice makes perfect' is all well and good, but perfect practice makes perfect is more to the point. Perfection in sport is virtually impossible, but the closer we are to being perfect the better we become, no matter the endeavour.

It leads us into the quality over quantity notion, where one hour of quality practice is better than three hours without much intent. Jack Nicklaus said he never hit a golf ball in practice without total focus and concentration on the task at hand. If true, I'm even more in awe of the Golden Bear because that's an incredibly tough thing to do. The message being, when you practise, treat each and every ball with the utmost commitment. It might be something technical in the swing, or a new shot you're learning, or perhaps a result-based game requiring PSR work. Whatever it is, if you strive for perfection, I guarantee you will get better. And when the real competition starts, your complete focus and concentration on the task at hand will become second nature.

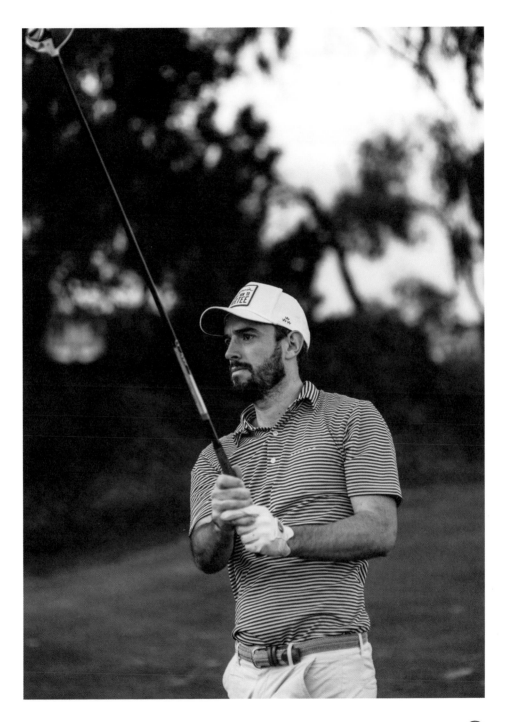

GSR:
Golf-Shot
Routine

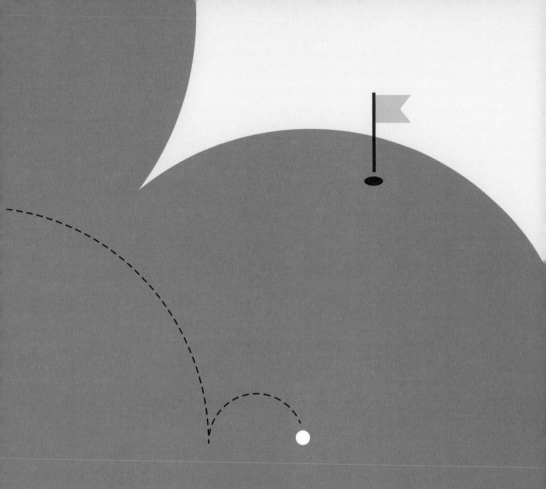

In *Tour Mentality*, I explained the principles and processes that laid the foundation to my mental game over the years. They revolve around a question I continually ask myself on the course: 'What do I have to do right now?' The answer is always the same: 'Stay in the present; commit to the process.'

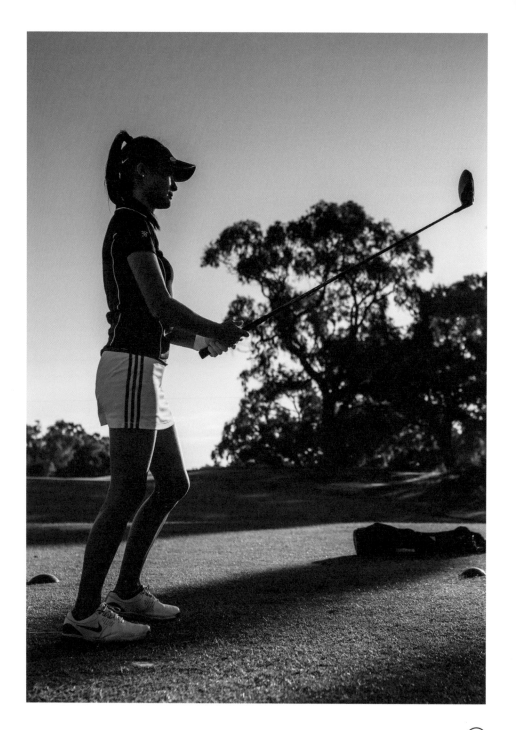

For each and every golf shot we need to bring our mind back to where it should be – in the now. Poor thinking occurs when thoughts drift into the past or future, typically result-based and not of a positive note. Once in the present moment, our focus is dictated by what's in front of us. At the ball, it's the **pre-shot routine (PSR)**, made up of two phases: **decide** and **execute**. Also included is a **precise target** and **acceptance** after the shot. If we're walking down the fairway, our intention is to **switch off**, and as we approach the ball, **switching on** comes into play. All these were my mental game foundations, and hopefully if you've read *Tour Mentality*, you've seen some benefits by implementing them into your games.

The most talked about is the **pre-shot routine**, however, **acceptance** and being able to **switch on** and especially **switch off** between shots are just as important. They are less obvious and, thus, the most neglected. In thinking about how to help golfers seamlessly include them for every shot, I've come up with the **golf-shot routine (GSR)**. First, let's quickly revisit each area.

Pre-Shot Routine (PSR)

Put simply, a PSR is the process for hitting a golf shot. It provides a focus and direction for our mind to follow. I like to think of my PSR as a protective bubble. After watching the Bubble Boy episode of *Seinfeld* many years ago, this protective bubble image gave me a sense of calm that nothing can penetrate the bubble (even though George did it in Seinfeld – lol). The PSR is divided up into two key phases.

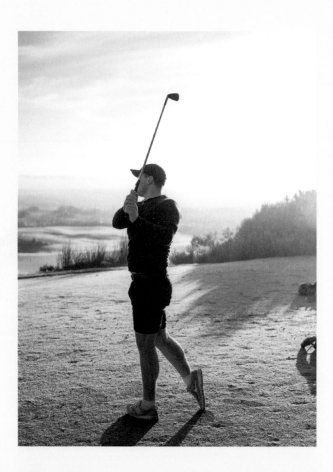

D

DECIDE (D)

The D phase takes place in the left side of the brain, where logic and thinking occur. We're gathering information for the shot at hand. For a full shot the lie, yardage, pin position, wind direction, slope, temperature, shot shape and so on all come into consideration (depending on how deep you want to go). Based on this information we make a decision, and most importantly, *commit* to this decision, so we don't start second-guessing ourselves in the next phase.

E

EXECUTE (E)*

The E phase occurs in the right side of the brain where creativity, sensing and feeling comes from. Peak performance resides here. When you hit your best golf shots you're not thinking, you're feeling. Tiger Woods says he loves the pressure moments because his senses become heightened. He doesn't think more, he feels more. An optimal E phase feels like you're on autopilot. It starts from when you stand behind the ball, and carries through to walking in and striking it. I even recommend timing how long it takes from your first step into the ball from behind, to getting comfortable over the ball, and hitting the shot. On average, I'm 12 seconds from start to finish here and that's about the norm. The idea is to be as consistent as possible with this time. I enjoy watching the end of tournaments on TV for this reason. When players speed up or take too long over the ball, poor shots usually follow. The best players follow the same routine. They control their time beautifully and have purpose to their process, resulting in quality shots more often than not.

PT

PRECISE TARGET (PT)

Aim small, miss small. When you lock in on a PT your bad shots become better. For example, on a tee shot, if your target is 'the fairway', a good shot finds the fairway and a bad shot doesn't. Whereas if you aim for a specific part of the fairway, a good shot goes exactly there, while the bad shot is perhaps still on the edge of the fairway rather than in the trees. Remember, golf isn't about the quality of your good shots, it's about the quality of your bad ones.

A

ACCEPTANCE (A)

How you react to the result of a shot has a profound influence on your attitude and mindset. There aren't many things you can control in golf. The PSR is one of them, and how you react to the result of a shot is another. Once the ball's gone you don't have any more say in it. However, you can control your reaction by *accepting* the result, good or bad. It's an invaluable skill. I'm all for having some sort of post-shot analysis, but don't dwell on it for too long – it's gone.

I worked with a talented young player a while ago who only saw the negative after every shot. Even after holing a nice putt he'd say, 'Well that's what I'm supposed to do.' I observed this for a few holes then gave him a goal to find something positive from each shot. On the next hole, a par five, he duffed his third shot straight into a greenside bunker and said sarcastically, 'So where's the positive in that?' I replied, 'Actually, you've missed the green in the perfect spot. It's a simple uphill bunker shot from there.' He mulled this over and must have agreed because his body language changed walking into the sand. He splashed the ball out into the hole for birdie. Simply by changing his attitude and accepting the result, his negativity wasn't carried over into the next shot. If he hadn't done this, bogey was almost a certainty.

---

*In *Tour Mentality*, I spoke about a 'swing thought' during the E phase. I've since realised a 'swing feel' might be more appropriate because a swing thought implies thinking. Now, I understand some golfers are more analytical in their approach to the game, so a swing thought may work better for them. Personally, I prefer a feel. The important thing is to keep it to only *one* 'swing feel' (or thought). Having multiple feels (or thoughts) during a one-second golf swing is not productive.

SWITCH ON, SWITCH OFF

(For some reason I've never abbreviated these)

Taking our mind away from the game between shots is one of the toughest things for golfers to do. We love thinking about what just happened and what might occur next. To help take my thoughts away from these scenarios I undo the velcro tab on my glove as a key to *switch off*. Then, I start chatting to my caddy or playing partners, or look at the trees, wildlife, anything to take my mind off golf. Approaching the ball, I use my glove again. Putting it back on is the signal to *switch on* and start narrowing my focus to the current situation. For putting, the act of walking onto the green is my *switch on* moment. While waiting for a playing partner to putt, I'll *switch off* briefly by looking around or taking a few deep breaths. It's only for a few moments, but it's better than thinking constantly on the green while waiting my turn.

AWARENESS

Finally, switching on and off starts with *awareness*. Being aware of thoughts helps redirect our mind to the present moment. As mentioned, I meditated throughout my career and it helped a great deal in making me aware of my thoughts. We all have negative thoughts; even the best players in the game have them. The key is to identify them and allow them to pass through without attachment. Meditation definitely helped with this. It gave me a sense of calm, so I never felt too anxious on the course. Sure, I still had some very intense moments, but they would have been more extreme without an awareness of them.

It's natural for the mind to wander from thought to thought during a round of golf. Scientists have shown we have around 70,000 thoughts a day. Since 18 holes can take four to five hours, we're well into that total number on the course. The skill is redirecting our mind to a thought appropriate for the moment. To do this, I ask myself, 'What do I have to do right now?'

Golf-Shot Routine (GSR)

Getting back to the GSR, here is the entire sequence from shot to shot broken down as follows:

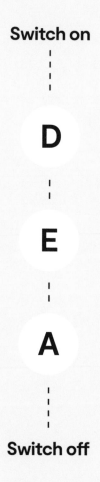

Switch on

D

E

A

Switch off

Approaching the ball, switch on by narrowing your focus to the shot at hand. Take in the necessary information, make a decision (D) and commit to it. Execute the shot (E), accept the result (A), and finally switch off. After a while, you approach the ball again, switch on and repeat the process.

If the average PSR takes around 30–40 seconds (from when we arrive at the ball to hitting it), the GSR will take about a minute, give or take. A few seconds before getting to the ball to switch on, 10–15 seconds after the shot to accept the result, and finally another few seconds to switch off. These times may vary, but they're a good baseline to start with. For putting, this time frame is shorter with tap-ins and so on. But for argument's sake, if we shoot 80, that's 80 minutes of GSRs out of a 240-minute round of golf. For the other 160 minutes we're enjoying the walk, talking to our playing partners or caddy, or simply looking at the wildlife on the course. The GSR provides a nice cushion either side of the PSR to ease in and out of. There you have it, a GSR! It probably won't catch on but it's my new acronym for the world of golf. ☺

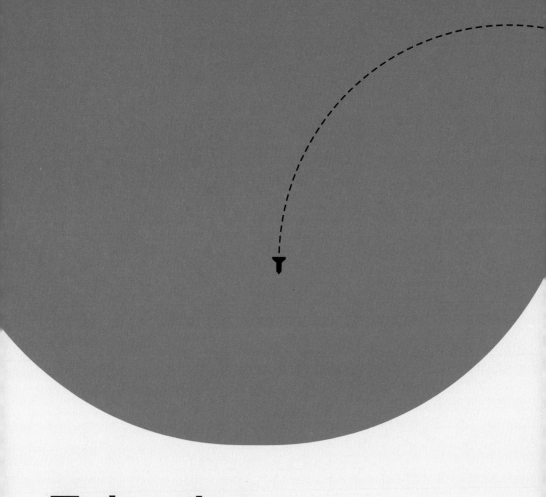

Take the Result Out of Play

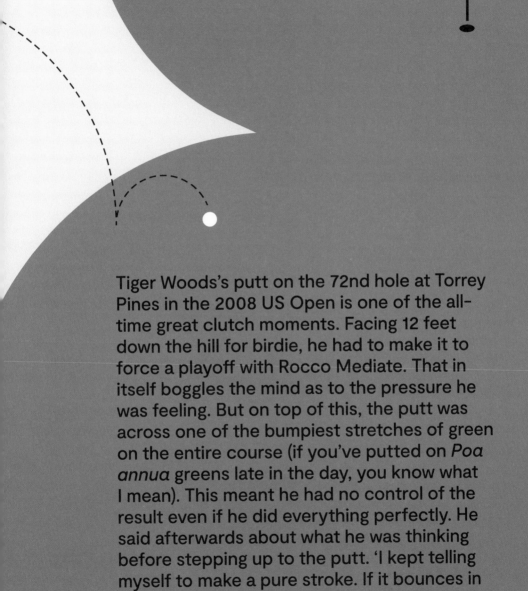

Tiger Woods's putt on the 72nd hole at Torrey Pines in the 2008 US Open is one of the all-time great clutch moments. Facing 12 feet down the hill for birdie, he had to make it to force a playoff with Rocco Mediate. That in itself boggles the mind as to the pressure he was feeling. But on top of this, the putt was across one of the bumpiest stretches of green on the entire course (if you've putted on *Poa annua* greens late in the day, you know what I mean). This meant he had no control of the result even if he did everything perfectly. He said afterwards about what he was thinking before stepping up to the putt. 'I kept telling myself to make a pure stroke. If it bounces in or out, so be it, at least I can hold my head up high if I make a pure stroke,' he said.

Given the magnitude of the occasion, having the presence of mind to bring his attention back to the process is why he's one of the greatest players in history. As his ball trundled down the slope, the crowd held its breath in anticipation, watching it bobble along the surface of the green. Finally, it fell in the right lip and the whole place went nuts. The following day he won in an extended playoff for his fourth US Open and 14th major title overall.

This incredible example leads me more into the nitty gritty of the PSR because, let's face it, this is where the magic happens. As discussed, there are two phases, D and E. Something I like helping golfers with is to *take the result out of play*. Usually, a slightly confused look comes across their face when I say this, so let's explore this statement.

The time to think about the result is during the D phase. In Tiger's case at Torrey Pines, it was while reading the green, evaluating the slope and break, and choosing a line. He was thinking about making it and the possibility of missing it too. It's okay to do the latter during the D phase. The key is to then focus on what gives you the best possible chance of executing the desired result. For Tiger, he knew this was to put a pure stroke on the ball. If he did that and it went in, great, and if not, well there's nothing more he could have done and he'd be okay with that. In essence, he took the result out of play and committed to the process.

Here's another example without a US Open title on the line for the rest of the 99.99 per cent of golfers out there. Halle's hit a nice drive on a par four and is left with a second shot to a green protected by water on the right-hand side. Her first thought is 'Don't hit it right in the water'. It's okay, get that thought out now during the D phase. It's part of the process. Perhaps going long is also a no-no, so she needs to take that into account as well. Having thought about where she *doesn't* want to hit it, she now focuses on where she *does* – perhaps 20 feet left and slightly short of the pin. Next, Halle calculates the necessary information applicable for this result – the lie, yardage, pin position, wind direction, shot shape, club selection and so on, depending on how in-depth she wants to go. This data helps her decide on the shot. She's thought about the result, both good and bad, come to a decision, and now commits to it. There's no need to focus on the result anymore because she's *taken it out of play*. Her attention now turns to the E phase.

This varies for golfers, but here's mine and it's a good template to work from:

1. Stand behind the ball and visualise the shot.

2. Take a practice swing feeling what's required to execute that shot.

3. Locate a precise target (PT).

4. Walk into the ball.

5. Focus on a swing feel.

6. React and let the shot go.

By moving through this process effortlessly the result takes care of itself. After a poor shot, I often hear golfers say, 'I was thinking about avoiding the trees on the right,' or 'I didn't want to skull it over the green,' or 'I was trying not to three-putt.' These are result-based thoughts that find their way into the E phase. They pop up because we're not fully committed to our decision in the D phase. There's doubt. About the decision, about our swing, or that the wind's blowing 30 km/h in our faces and creating problems. Fine, let's back away and re-evaluate until we come to a fully committed decision. Anything less and the process will likely break down. Because let's face it, when was the last time you hit a good shot while in a poor state of mind over the ball? Ultimately, we have to back ourselves.

Once committed, the E phase should feel like being on autopilot (we're in the right half of our brain, the creative, sensing, feeling side). All thinking has been done already (in the logical left side). If a thought occurs about what might happen or happened previously, back away and start again. Our goal is to be consistent in our movements (how many steps into the ball, looks at the target, waggles and so forth) and time frame (how long it takes from when you take your first step to the ball from behind to hitting the shot). Every so often, for example, I time this part of my putting E phase over 10 tries with a stopwatch (it's 12 seconds). I want consistent movements and times (typically within half a second for each try). It's my comfort zone for every shot on the course because I control this time. After the ball leaves the putter face, whatever happens is up to the golfing gods. Same goes for the full swing, chipping, bunker shots and all the rest.

When we play our best golf, we're not worried about where the ball's going while over the ball. There's no thinking, just feeling and reacting to the shot. We've committed to the shot and *taken the result out of play*. If we follow this process, the result will take care of itself.

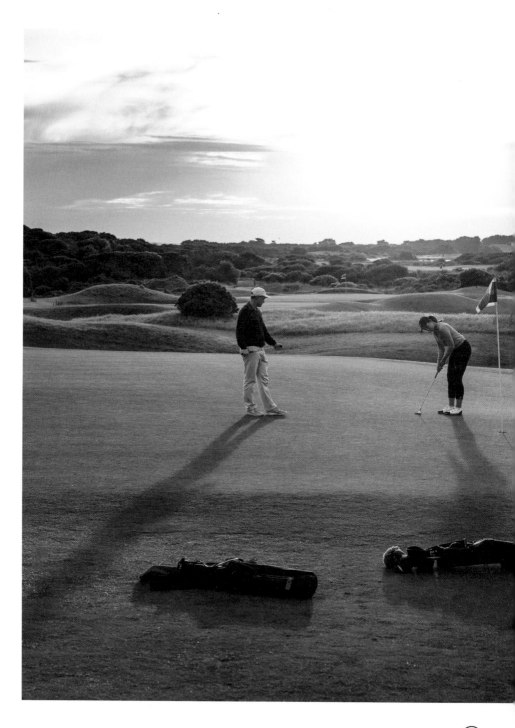

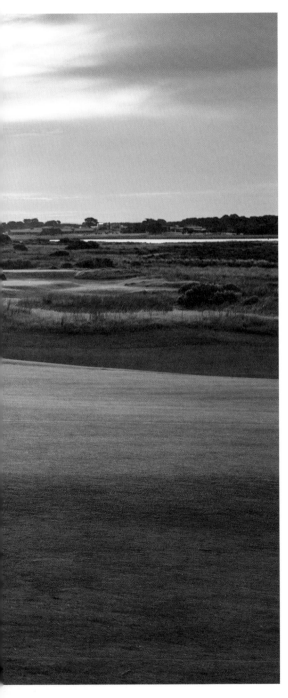

' When we play our best golf, we're not worried about where the ball's going while over the ball. There's no thinking, just feeling and reacting to the shot.'

The Hardest Thing About Golf

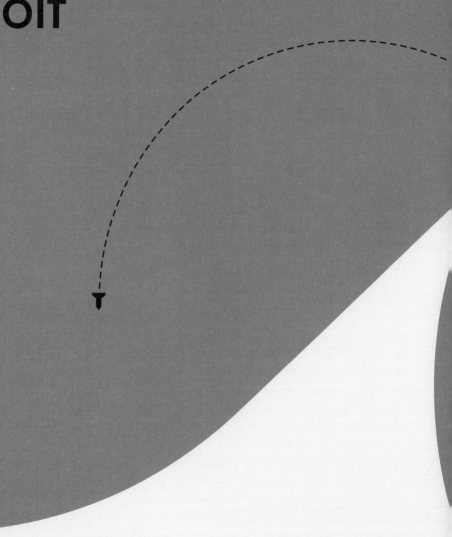

I alluded to this earlier, and after playing and coaching golfers for many years, one of the hardest things about this game is that the ball is stationary. For this reason, I believe golf is the most mentally challenging sport. I'm sure elite athletes from other sports will disagree, but golf is unique because we have to create the ball's movement when standing over it, plus there is so much time to think about everything between shots. For just about every other sport, the ball is moving, so you are reacting to it. In golf we generate the ball's movement. That, plus all that time to think, allows moments for doubt and indecision to creep in.

The most mentally challenging moments in other sports are when the ball is at rest, or the athlete has to initiate movement. For example, penalty kicks in soccer, field goals (and extra point conversions) in the NFL, rugby, and set shots on goal in Aussie rules football (also known as AFL), to name a few. I've noticed an increasing trend of late in the AFL where players kicking set shots for goal are resorting to a 'hook' method. They feel more comfortable doing this because it feels like a kick in the run of play. Perhaps the indignation of missing a relatively straightforward set shot on goal has forced them to try this method, instead of refining and improving the process of a uniform attempt. It would be exciting to work with athletes in these different sporting codes to help them develop a productive 'pre-kick routine' much like a golfer's PSR. They'd just call it a PKR instead. ☺

A way to make a golf shot more reactive is by taking less time from when you bring your eyes back to the ball after the last look at the target to starting the swing. This goes for all shots, full swings, chipping, bunker shots and putting. The longer we dwell over the ball after our last look at the target, the more time there is for us to think about things. Have a think about what your good days feel like, and I bet you don't spend too much time over the ball. First, you see the shot, walk in, get comfortable and simply react. On bad days the opposite is true. We're indecisive, we take too long over the ball and our rhythm suffers. Our minds tick away worrying where the ball might go, or about our swing. The 'what ifs' occur. What if this happens? What if I do that? These days are mentally draining; believe me, I've been there. Another positive to reacting to the ball is it promotes rhythm in the swing, or rhythm in the stroke for a putt. But more on this shortly. For now, focus on reacting more to the target, and I guarantee you'll have better rhythm and a freedom that makes the game more enjoyable.

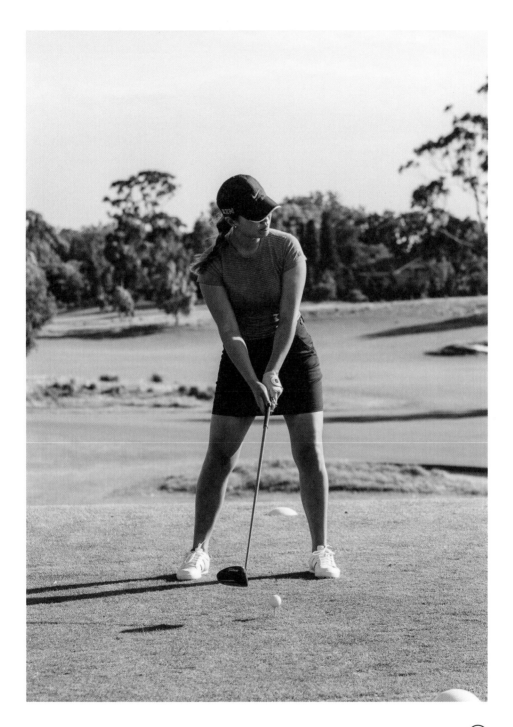

The Hardest Thing About Golf

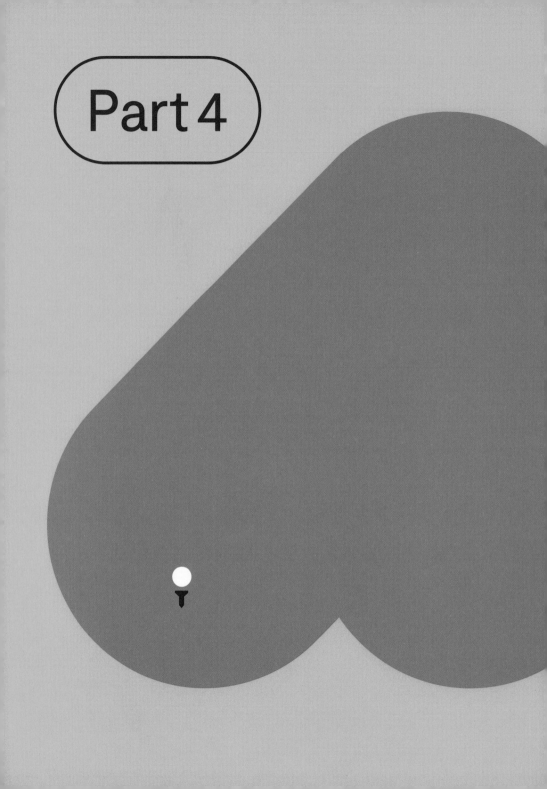

Part 4

The Scoring Clubs

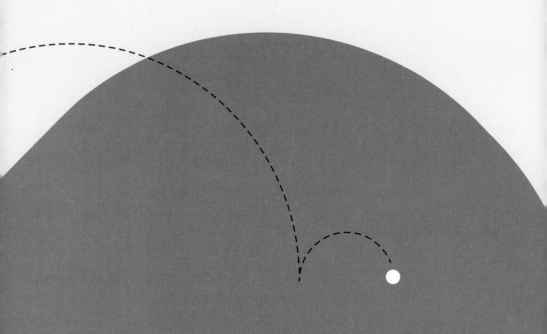

Putting:
Rhythm
and Tempo

People often ask me who I enjoyed playing with on tour. If my name was next to Ernie Els, Nick Faldo or Michael Campbell on the time sheet I was a happy camper. The reason? They all had incredible rhythm and tempo in their games, which seemed to rub off on me. I think the worst score I shot playing with Ernie was five under. His nickname, the 'Big Easy' sums up his nature (even though he's as competitive as anyone), and how he plays is hypnotic. Watching Faldo hit balls in his heyday was observing a master at his craft. Where others looked to the technical simplicity of his swing, I enjoyed the overall flow. Playing with Nick was never a chatty affair though, as he was always totally dedicated to the task at hand. 'Play well' and 'Thanks for the game' was about all you got out of him over the four or five hours on the course. Cambo's game is poetry in motion and fun to watch when on a hot streak. Unfortunately, I was on the wrong end of one when, as my playing partner in the final group, he shot 64 on Sunday one year at the Heineken Classic in Perth to win comfortably.

From a putting perspective I love playing with Brad Faxon. His silky smooth stroke and reputation as one of the best putters in the world is well warranted. The way the ball rolls off his putter seems like it almost has no choice but to fall in the hole. His stroke has an effortless 'catch and shoot' (in basketball terms) look to it, but believe me, he worked his arse off for it to appear this way. From all my years watching and playing with the best putters in the world, the common traits they all possess are great rhythm and tempo.

What are rhythm and tempo when it comes to putting? Rhythm is the relationship between backswing to forward swing speed, while tempo is the time it takes from the start of your stroke to impact. I believe the tempo is determined by your personality, As I mentioned in the opening chapter, the type of golfer you are should reflect your personality 'Play like your personality' (page 14). In this case, for an upbeat, hyper person with quicker tendencies, their putting stroke should follow suit. For an easygoing, relaxed, take-your-time type, ideally that's reflected in their stroke too.

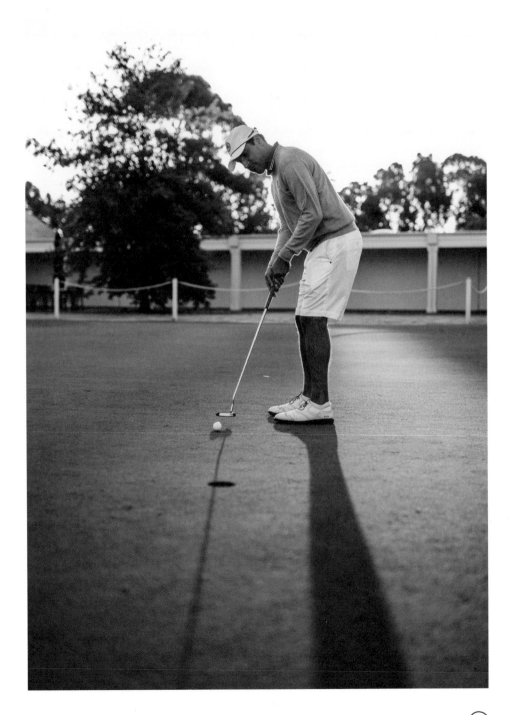

To help my putting rhythm and tempo, I use a counting method when practising. It was first brought to my attention by Steve Bann, an Australian teaching pro who's helped various top players over the years: Ian Baker-Finch, Stuart Appleby, Robert Allenby, KJ Choi and Danny Lee to name a few. We were discussing putting one day and he mentioned Kel Nagle (one of the all-time great putters) used a simple counting method like this:

1   **He placed the putter head in front of the ball (an old-school tendency not seen anymore).**

2   **He moved the putter head back behind the ball.**

3   **He looked at the target.**

4   **He brought his eyes back to the ball.**

5   **He started the stroke.**

I've shortened this method to 1 - 2 - 3, the equivalent of Kel's 3 - 4 - 5. Whether it's fast or slow (tempo) is up to the individual (depending on their personality), it's the timing (rhythm) that needs to be consistent. By this I mean each number coming at the same pace.

E.g.

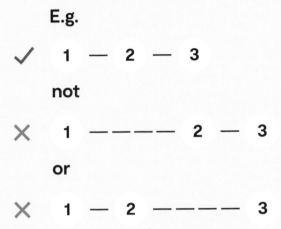

Use a metronome (try between 70 and 80 bpm as a guide) or find a song that has a nice beat. Both do wonders for your putting stroke in the rhythm and tempo departments.

A quicker count (1-2-3) will result in a shorter, faster stroke (quicker tempo). Players such as Brandt Snedeker or Stacy Lewis are like this. A slower count (1 -- 2 -- 3) produces a longer, smoother stroke (slower tempo). Think Loren Roberts or Inbee Park. I'm between both with a 1 - 2 - 3 count.

You can also experiment with adding in the number 4, which comes at the moment contact is made with the ball. This seems to help some players and it goes like this:

1   Look at the target.

2   Bring your eyes back to the ball.

3   Start the stroke.

4   Make contact with the ball.

The counting method has two benefits. Firstly, it improves distance control because our rhythm and tempo are better. A vital part of putting is to *react* to the putt rather than *think* about it. Golfers struggle with their speed and distance control when they pause too long over the ball. They lose their feel for the putt, tense up, and the stroke suffers. The counting helps the overall flow to the routine.

Secondly, it also takes our mind away from the result, especially on shorter putts. Short putts are more a mental challenge because the result is right there in front of us. We should make it and as a result our stroke suffers from tension by being too quick, or decelerating and so on. How many times have you put a good stroke on a 3-footer and it hasn't gone in? Rarely, I'm sure, and if it does miss, what more could you have done anyway? Perhaps you misread it, or the ball took a bobble on the way to the hole. That's golf, it happens, and I can live with those things. A poor stroke, however, I'm not happy about. By counting 1 - 2 - 3 on shorter putts you forget about the hole.

Our goal over every putt is to roll the ball well on the intended line with good speed. To do this we need to:

a. commit to the read and

b. put the best stroke on it possible.

By doing both of these well, the chances of making the putt go up enormously. I putt my best when I don't care if I make or miss it. I simply focus on being committed and a pure stroke.

I remember Brad Faxon saying that after having 35 putts one day. Someone said it was a shame he didn't putt well. Brad said, 'What do you mean I didn't putt well? I rolled the ball beautifully today. They just didn't go in.' That's the mindset of a great putter. His focus was on the process and if he continually executed that in the correct fashion, the ball will start to drop at some stage. On this particular day, it just wasn't to be. I'm sure the following day was a different story.

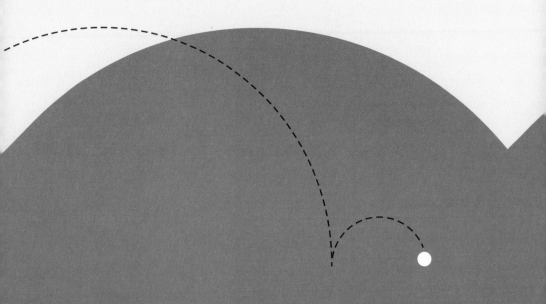

Putting:
Speed
Determines
the Line

Most three-putts occur because of poor speed, not poor line. Think about it: how often are you 3 feet (or more) wide of the hole on a 30-foot putt, compared to 3 feet (or more) short or long? To me, speed is more important than line and, thus, speed determines the line. If you had perfect speed every time during a round of golf, how would you putt? You wouldn't three-putt, have plenty of tap ins, and make more from longer distance because the hole becomes bigger with good speed.

Imagine three golf balls rolling side by side toward a hole. If your speed is too fast, only the middle ball goes in, the other two lip out. Too soft and obviously none go in. With good speed all three balls can find their way to the bottom of the cup by using all 4¼ inches. Inbee Park on the LPGA Tour is one of the best putters in the world. She has beautiful speed to her putts and it's no coincidence her tempo is on the slow side. Golfers with faster tempos are more aggressive putters. Those with a slower tempo tend to die their putts around the hole thus giving themselves more chance for putts to fall in.

Speed is based on feel, touch, instinct. We all have it, we just need to tap into it. When someone says they have no feel or touch, I ask them to underarm a ball to me on the full from 10 feet away. After catching it and tossing it back, I move 5 feet further away and ask them to do the same. Again, I catch it and move further back. Typically, after doing this a few times at varying distances they're able to toss me the ball so I catch it each time on the full. I ask them, 'How did you know how far to toss the ball to me?' They reply, 'I don't know, I just threw it.' That's feel, instinct. They weren't thinking, 'Okay, Nick's 25 feet away so I need to pull my arm back 180 degrees and accelerate through at 6 mph.' No, they just saw I moved further away and reacted. They already have the necessary feel – they just don't quite know how to translate it to putting.

As mentioned, a stationary ball is what makes golf hard. If it was moving, there'd be less thinking, instinct would take over and you would simply react. It's why I like the counting method. It helps me react to the target, allowing instinct to take over, thus producing good speed. To exaggerate this even further, try hitting putts by starting the stroke 'before' your eyes come back to the ball. It has that 'catch and shoot' feel like Brad Faxon has.

When someone has a 15-foot putt with right-to-left break, they ask, 'How much break do you think there is?' I always reply, 'It depends on your speed.' With dying speed there's more break, with firmer speed less break. I don't know how hard they are going to hit the putt. I only sense how hard I would hit it. So, I say, 'It's around 2 to 3 feet right to left depending on your speed', then leave it up to them. I don't use a line on my ball for this reason. It predetermines the speed and takes the feel out of it. The same goes for the line I'm seeing. It's not an exact, thin line, rather a wide shaded path about the width of a hole. I'll talk more about this in the next chapter on reading greens (page 164).

The final ingredient for good speed is to have the backswing and follow-through match in length. How far you take the putter head back is how far you should take it through. Now, there are always exceptions to the rule, Ben Crenshaw comes to mind here. He had quite a long backswing and a shorter follow-through. He also had incredible feel and touch, making him one of the greatest putters of all time. In general, though, for better consistency with speed I've found having the backswing and follow-through match up in length the best formula. On shorter putts, the backswing and follow-through are shorter, while on longer putts they are obviously longer. Tempo determines how far back and through your putter head will travel as well. A slower tempo means a longer backswing and follow-through. A faster tempo equates to a shorter backswing and follow-through.

The beauty about having good speed is you don't need to be as precise with the line because the hole becomes bigger. You'll rarely three-putt and have plenty of tap-ins. It will help you be more relaxed on the greens, and that's a really cool state to be in with a putter in hand.

Drill

Leapfrog: Find a flat area on a practice green and drop five balls down as your starting point. Walk five paces (about 15 feet) and place a coin on the ground. Step another three paces and put a tee in the ground. These are your front and back markers (about 9 feet apart). The goal is to roll the five balls between the coin and the tee, each ball past the previous one, hence leapfrog. If you're short of the previous ball or past the back tee, start again. Don't worry about aim, all you're doing is controlling distance. Once you complete five balls in a row, take a step back to six paces (18 feet) from the coin and repeat, then seven paces and so on, until eventually you're 10 paces (30 feet) away from the coin. After a while you'll know instantly whether a putt is short, good or too long. Vary the difficulty depending on your skill level. Start with three balls, then progress to four and finally five. Change the slope to uphill, downhill, left to right and right to left. It's a great drill to quickly adjust to the speed of a course's greens because typically a golf club's practice green is similar to what's out on the course. There are a variety of speed drills, but this is my favourite.

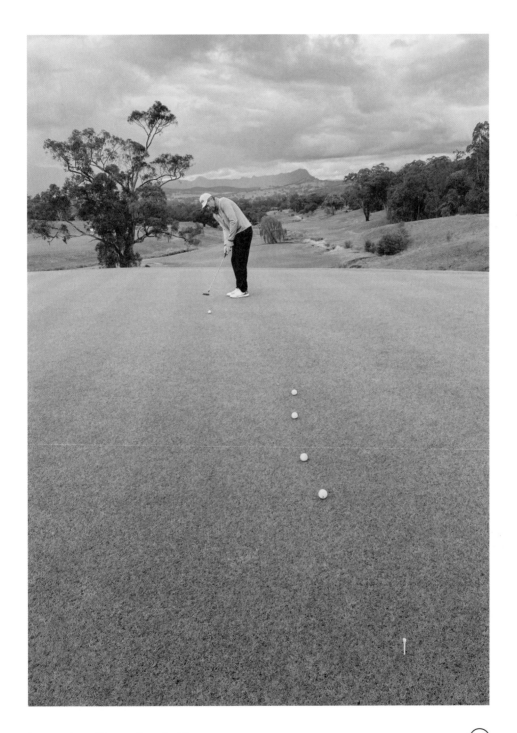

Putting: Speed Determines the Line

Putting: the Art of Reading Greens

For me, green reading is an art form; for some, it's a science. In my experience, scientists can be good putters, but the great ones are artists. Opinions vary, but, as always, find what works best for you. There are several important things to consider as we walk onto a green and begin the challenge of reading a putt.

Think about this: have you ever stood to the side watching your playing partner putt, and as their ball is rolling toward the hole, you know whether it's going in or not? It's amazing how you can tell the result from the side and be right nine times out of 10. That's the first aspect to reading greens – look from the side, not just from behind. Ideally the low side as it provides the best view on the overall break and slope. On a left-to-right putt, look from the right, the low side.

Here's an example of how most golfers read putts. They walk straight over to the ball, mark, clean and replace it, take a look from behind, and move into the putt. It gives them a general sense of things, but really they're only halfway to knowing what the read is. I understand golfers want to keep pace of play moving, but we can ascertain a lot about a putt by being more observant as we walk to our ball, and even from back in the fairway. We can see things from a distance that sometimes we don't see from right on top. As we walk onto a green, start by taking in the green's overall tilt. Does it slant from back to front, left to right? Are there any tiers or drop-offs? Where would water drain off in a heavy downpour? This is a great indicator as to a green's overall slope. If possible, walk by the hole to see what's happening around there. This is where the putt will break the most as it slows down.

If we have time, take a stroll around the entire line to see it from all angles. The slopes become more obvious and we may notice the ball breaks two different ways or straightens up in certain areas. This can also be felt in our feet walking around. Reading greens isn't just about what we see but what we feel. Not that I've tried it, but I assume the AimPoint method is based on this because AimPoint players use their feet as a gauge for slope. By feeling the slopes as we walk, bending down to take a closer look sometimes isn't necessary. When I played the first two rounds with Ben Crenshaw at The Masters one year, this was his style. He'd walk around the entire putt, get a feel for it, move into the ball and stroke it. He wouldn't bend down for a closer look, instead he simply trusted his instincts. To my recollection, he never missed a putt inside 10 feet and it remains one of the greatest putting displays I've ever seen.

For longer and/or uphill putts there won't be much break at the start because in the first part of its journey a ball's speed negates the break (unless it's severe). The last half of the putt is where break comes more into it, as the ball starts slowing down. Look around the hole. It's an excellent guide to what part of the hole the ball will best fall in given the slope and break. Work backwards from there to find the path the ball needs to take. Speed determines the line and on longer putts it's crucial for the line we take. Visualise an overall path too. As mentioned, I'm not one for seeing an exact line, more a wider path (about hole width) to roll my ball on. This image frees me up because I'm not worried about hitting my ball on the perfect line. Being too precise creates tension in the hands, resulting in a poor stroke. If you watch tournaments on TV, you'll see on longer putts an overlaid shaded area on the green in their graphics. It expands and shrinks on the ball's journey to the hole, showing the various lines a putt can be rolled on, depending on speed. For very short putts, we can almost take break out of the equation by being quite firm. This requires confidence and belief in our stroke because the hole gets smaller the firmer the putt is struck – but it does make them a lot straighter. Tiger Woods in his heyday putted this way.

Another important element is grain and the type of grass we're putting on. The most common varieties on greens are Bermuda, Bent and *Poa annua*. Bermuda greens are the grainiest and it's clearly detectable. Look from the ball to the hole and if the grass is shiny or lighter in colour, the grain is going away from you, therefore the putt is quicker and breaks more. Darker, duller grass shows you're into the grain, so it's a slower putt with less break. Typically, the grain follows the slope, so downhill/down grain and uphill/into the grain ring true. On sidehill putts such as a right-to-left putt with the grain following the slope, break is emphasised, so allow a bit more. The trickiest reads on grainy greens are the subtle ones where there isn't much slope or break. It may look like the ball wants to move right, yet the grain's going left. Taking these both into account combined with speed provides the correct answer. On these I recommend walking around the entire line for a good sense of the read.

Bent greens don't have as much grain but can still have some effect. The shades of lighter and darker grass on Bent is more subtle than Bermuda, but it's the best way to determine if there's any grain. Augusta National's Bent greens are some of the quickest I've putted on anywhere in the world. Mostly because the severe slopes magnify the speed, to ridiculous proportions at times. I've had 10-foot downhill putts at The Masters where all I'm thinking is, 'How can I 2-putt from here?' That's where the artistry comes in (watch Ben Crenshaw). Greens on Melbourne's sandbelt courses are just as quick and some of the purest to putt on if you get the chance; to name a few: Royal Melbourne, Kingston Heath, Metropolitan, Victoria. They are the ultimate examination in speed, green reading and touch.

Poa annua greens are an interesting proposition because they change as the day goes on. Other types of grass can too, but the seed heads of *Poa* become larger as the grass grows, meaning the greens get bumpier as the day wears on. Pebble Beach's *Poa* greens have worn out many a player's patience at the AT&T tournament. Nicely struck 3-footers don't even touch the hole late in the day there.

As grasses and maintenance improve each year, different strains come out smoother and more resistant to weather. Greens keep getting better, but the art of reading them remains unchanged. On tour they used to go down the scientific route with green-reading books showing the direction, gradient and degree of slopes for each section of a green. It takes away some of the skill and slows up play. Players would stand there looking at the book and all I could think was, 'Look at the green, not the book!' I'd always thought the governing bodies should ban them and at the end of 2021, they did. If you have to rely on them, you probably don't have the best feel and touch anyway. I've never seen Tiger Woods, Ben Crenshaw or Brad Faxon use a green-reading book, so that tells us all something.

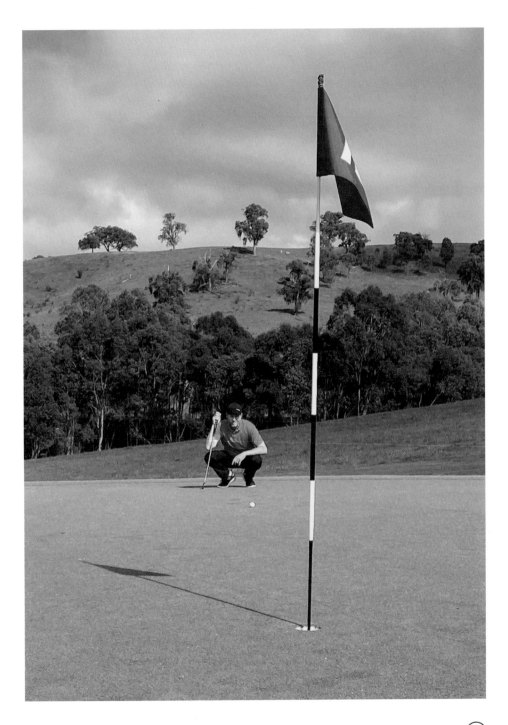

Putting: the Art of Reading Greens

Wind can have an effect especially on greens exposed to the elements. Exceptionally strong winds have even halted play at tournaments because balls won't stop moving on the greens. These days are rare, but factoring wind into the speed and break on putts is important. A left-to-right putt with the wind blowing from the right can get very interesting. How much the putt's affected is a judgement call based on feel. On windy days rhythm and tempo are the primary focus for a solid strike. Miss-hit putts veer off-line in an exaggerated fashion, much like miss-hit full shots in the wind. I enjoy practising on windy days to figure out these scenarios, along with how much to widen my stance for stability.

Moisture is another consideration for reading putts. Early morning dew slows putts down and reduces the amount of break. Sometimes in the morning you can see the line a previous player's ball took. It's a nice pre-read and can help you to visualise your own line – although it doesn't tell you how hard they hit it. As the dew burns off, putts become quicker and begin to break more. Rain has a similar effect, slowing putts down and creating less turn. Shorter putts become quite straight allowing you to be firmer knowing the ball won't go too far past.

As you can see, there's plenty of information to absorb and interpret when reading greens. It all starts as we approach the green from the fairway, and by opening up our senses we get an overall feel for what the green does before we even reach our ball. Remember, reading greens is fun. When you enjoy the challenge of solving each putt, you'll love walking onto a green.

Drill

Vacant hole: Ideally, this drill is done on a quiet practice putting green. For example, if there are 5 vacant holes, start at one hole and drop four balls down. Putt one ball to each of the 4 vacant holes and hole them out. Then putt each ball back to the original hole you started at, totalling 8 holes. Four out, four in. Every hole is a par two. Keep score, move to the next hole and repeat. If you have time, do this for all 5 holes, but even just a couple is fine. Every putt is different (like out on the course), so reading each one is important. It helps you quickly dial in the speed and slopes, plus the competitive element (hole vs hole score) makes it interesting.

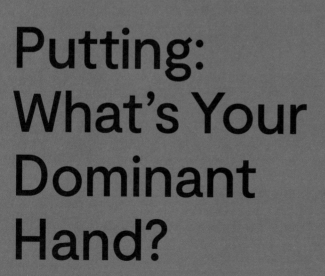

Putting:
What's Your
Dominant
Hand?

A dominant eye is talked about in golf and sport, but for me, a dominant hand is just as important when it comes to putting. I like to joke I've made the biggest change in the history of putting, going from a long left-handed putter to a regular length right-handed one. You can't get a much bigger change than that! Throughout my career I used a 48-inch left-handed broomstick putter. When the anchoring rule was introduced a few years ago, I found un-anchoring the long putter a struggle, so I began the search for an alternative. I tried a regular length left-handed putter using several grip variations without success, then a slightly longer putter with the armlock method most famously used by Matt Kuchar. It worked for a while but never felt very comfortable. By the way, how this is not anchoring is beyond me.

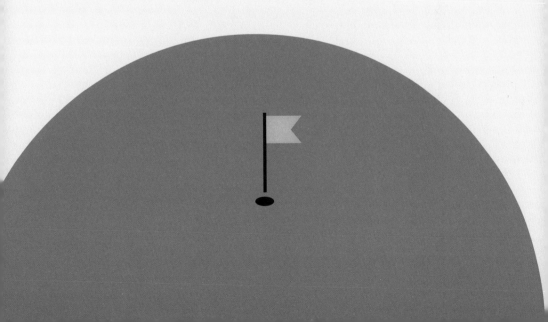

Then one day the magic happened by chance. For fun, I played the front 9 holes at Isleworth right-handed to see what I could shoot. After a couple of lost balls and some mistakes here and there, I shot 48, but what surprised me was I only had 15 putts. I was amazed how good my feel and touch were. Walking onto greens was actually enjoyable. Pondering this afterwards, it suddenly made sense. I'm naturally right-handed with one-handed activities like writing, throwing a ball and playing tennis. If I rolled a ball to a hole with my hand, I'd use my right hand, not the left. So, putting from the right side felt completely natural.

To begin, the hardest part was aiming. Being so used to seeing putts from a left-handed perspective (looking to the right), turning my head the other way (to the left) felt totally foreign. Over time this adjustment became easier, but even to this day I still can't tell you exactly where I'm aiming on a 10-foot putt. The best part is that it doesn't matter. My feel and instinct for the speed and line take over, and I'm putting with more freedom than ever.

Initially, the most logical thing to do was put a line on the ball to help with aim. But I found it made me think about speed rather than feel it, so I abandoned that quickly. A lot of tour pros use a line, and I'm not saying it's a bad thing, it's just not for me. Try both, with and without a line, and see which works for you. One of the players I help uses the line for shorter putts, within 6 feet give or take, where speed doesn't play as big a part. Anything outside that range, he doesn't use the line and goes by feel. Personally, I think the line should be banned. It's a guide for alignment, something not allowed in golf, and aiming is a skill. Again, that's for another discussion, but at least they banned caddies lining up their players on tour. I mean, come on, that's ridiculous!

Since making the switch to right-handed, my stats are very similar to the peak years I had on tour using the left-handed broomstick. The biggest difference is that I've gone back to putting more like an artist than a scientist. Whenever I struggled on the greens, the mistake I made was trying to 'science' the solution rather than relying on my artistic side. Putting right-handed has triggered that creativity again and I love walking onto a green now and seeing what challenge lies ahead. It's all to do with my dominant hand.

Remember, putting is a completely different game to the full swing. One is played along the ground, the other through the air. It shouldn't matter how you do it or what you look like. I've had plenty of strange looks and sometimes people don't even realise I'm putting the opposite way. After 9 holes they say, 'Hang on, you're putting right-handed!' I just laugh and start explaining why. If you're struggling with putting, try this. Roll a ball to a hole with your hand. Do you naturally use your right or left hand — and do you play golf this way? If it's the opposite, don't be afraid to give putting a go from this side and have some fun. I certainly am.

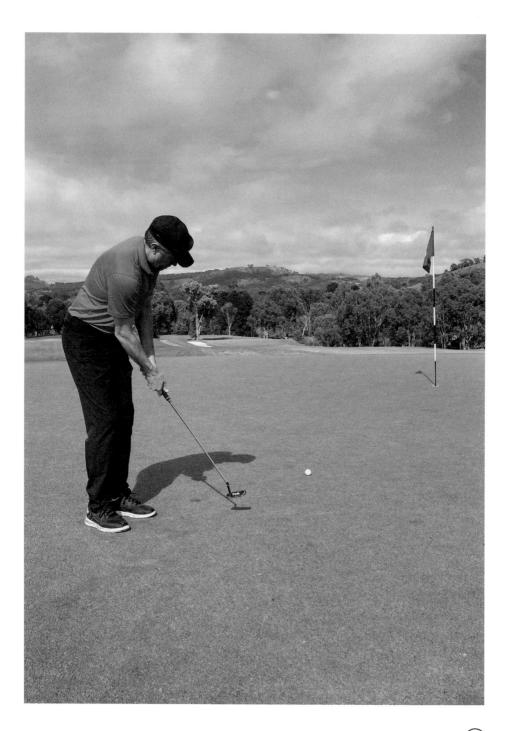

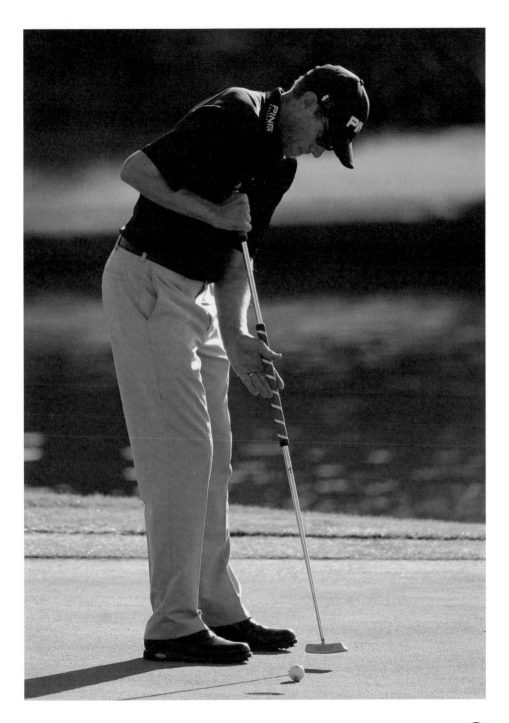

Putting: What's Your Dominant Hand?

The Importance of Wedges

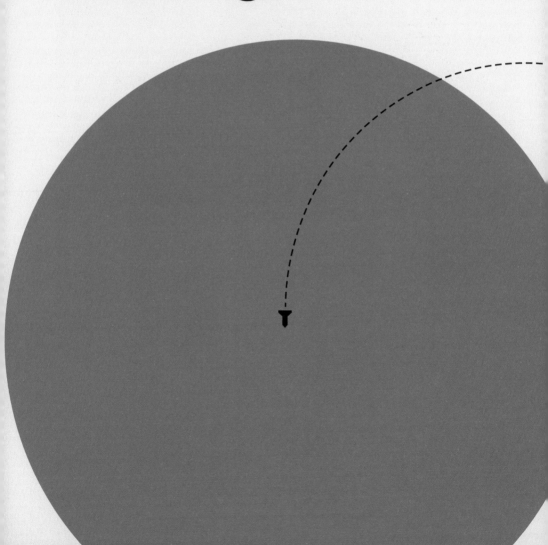

I played with Dustin Johnson early in his career and the talent was obvious. My lasting impression was once he figured out how to control wedges, he could become the best player in the world. Obviously, he knew that too and went to work on them with Butch Harmon and has since had incredible success. His wedge play is now a strength rather than a weakness. Wedges are our scoring clubs, or perhaps I should say our scoring distance clubs because wedge distance is where we can shave strokes off our score immediately. Good wedge play involves controlling distance and spin.

I have three wedges, a 46-degree pitching wedge (PW), 54-degree gap wedge (GW) and 60-degree lob wedge (LW). These lofts may differ for you, and many golfers have four wedges with lofts being, for example, 48, 52, 56 and 60 degrees. Whatever's in your bag, the goal is to control the distance and spin for each effectively. Direction isn't as big a deal, since they are easier to hit straight. However, if you are missing greens left or right, then obviously some work there is still needed. Interestingly, I find golfers get more upset when they hit a shot 20-feet pin high left or right, than one straight at the flag but 30 feet long or short. They feel the latter are better shots, which makes no sense.

Controlling distance and spin comes down to how hard we hit the shot and the angle of attack into the ball. The harder we hit a wedge the more spin it creates and the less control we have. Coming into the ball at a steeper angle has a similar affect. Golfers tend to get steep because the ball is too far back in the stance. Aim for middle – even a touch forward of middle promotes a shallower angle of attack so the leading edge digs less.

I have three different swings for my wedges – half, three-quarters and full swing. I relate these to a clockface, something Dave Pelz mentions in his *Short Game Bible*. It's not an exact science for me like Pelz professes, more a feeling, but the clockface is a nice mental image. For a right-handed golfer the backswing length with the left arm is 9 o'clock for the half swing, 10 o'clock for the three-quarter swing and 11 o'clock for the full swing. Also, I feel my follow-through length matches the backswing length, whereas Pelz likes a full follow-through for all of them. Each to their own.

My stock carry distances for each wedge and swing are as follows:

	60-degree	54-degree	46-degree
Half-swing	55 yards/ 50 metres	71 yards/ 65 metres	82 yards/ 75 metres
Three-quarter swing	71 yards/ 65 metres	87 yards/ 80 metres	104 yards/ 95 metres
Full swing	85 yards/ 78 metres	104 yards/ 95 metres	125 yards/ 115 metres

These distances relate to a normal day weather-wise. If it's cold, hot, raining or at altitude, then these can vary a few metres up or down.

A full swing is just your normal swing — simple. For a three-quarter swing, take a little off the length of that. Same again for the half swing. But control the backswing length through the turn of the body (don't just shorten your arm swing) with your arms staying connected. Interestingly, the half swing can take the longest to become consistent with because it's tougher to feel how long the backswing should be. The shot comes out lower, has less spin, takes more bounces and rolls out further. Having three different wedge swings is more for elite players and avid golfers. What I highly recommend though for all golfers is a three-quarter swing for each wedge. It's the easiest to control distance and spin with.

Dialling these in can be done a few different ways. The most common now is with a TrackMan (or similar device) that measures various numbers including carry distance. For example, hit 10 balls with a 60-degree lob wedge using a three-quarter swing. Eliminate the shots that aren't hit solid (thinned or chunked shots) and average out the carry distances of the rest. If you don't have a TrackMan, another way is hitting shots to pre-measured targets. Originally, I did it by having my caddy, Wilbur, stand out on the range shagging balls. He'd hold fingers up telling me how close I was to a particular yardage. Once these are under control, you'll find a favourite yardage and club after a while. Mine was a three-quarter 54-degree gap wedge around the 87-yard (80-metre) mark. I'd lay up as close to that number as often as I could on par fives or short par fours.

With the half and three-quarter swings the set-up changes slightly. For the half swing, narrow the stance quite a bit, aim a little left of target, open up your left foot a touch and lean your weight into your left side as you would for a long chip or pitch shot. Instead of using your hands to release the club through the ball, feel your arms and body (trunk) stay connected. The turn of the body (pivot) is what provides control and consistency. The three-quarter swing set-up is in between that and the full swing set-up. Because the swing is slightly longer you will feel a little more release of the hands. However, the turn through the ball and connection of hands, arms and body is what provides the control. Hitting half and three-quarter shots from a full swing set-up makes solid contact difficult and takes the feel out of the shot.

Some of the best wedge players I've come across include Steve Stricker, David Toms, Tim Clark and Luke Donald, to name a few. Steve and David have ideal full swings that translate beautifully for wedges. Their swings are wide with not much wrist hinge, promoting a shallow angle of attack. Both are incredible at controlling distance and spin. Tim and Luke worked their butts off with wedges – it looked as though they were throwing darts with them at times. When Luke reached No. 1 in the world his proximity to hole (PTH) was unbelievable and well ahead of the next best player. Combined with phenomenal putting, you'd back him, more often than not, to get it up and down with a wedge.

Try to avoid maxing out a wedge, meaning to hit it as hard as possible. They are very tough to control unless you hit them perfectly. The only time I'd max out a wedge is to an extremely firm green requiring lots of spin to hold it, or a front pin where the only way to get it close is by spinning the ball back to it. In that sense, for elite players you can have a fourth swing, on top of the half, three-quarter and full swings, called a 'max' swing. It may go 5 yards or so further than your full swing, but only use it when you have to. I'd much rather hit a three-quarter pitching wedge than a maxed-out gap wedge because the former is more consistent.

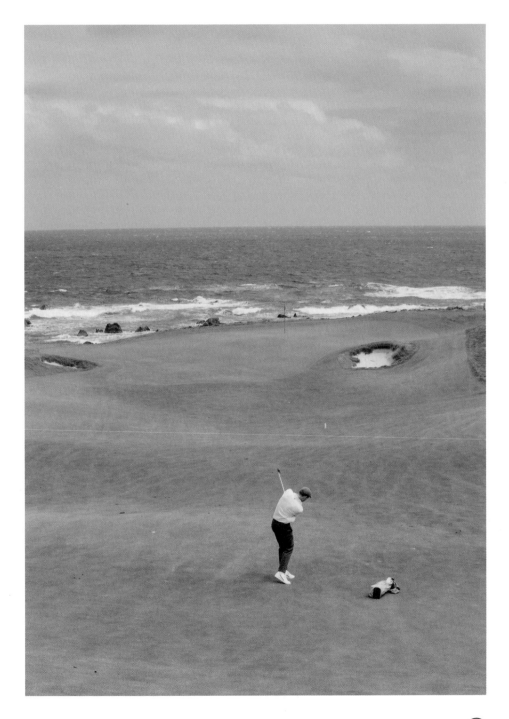

Drill

Wedge ball: On the course drop a ball at wedge distance out from each green and play it as a par two. For golfers with a lower skill level call it a par three. Over 9 holes I play the wedge ball from random distances on each hole, making sure I use my lob, gap and pitching wedges three times each, adding up to nine wedge shots. The goal (as a par two), and depending on conditions, is to shoot +6 or better for 9 holes, or getting up and down at least three out of nine times.

For the wedge ball drill on the opposite page, write down the proximity to hole (PTH) for each shot. Add those distances up at the end and average out the total number for your average PTH. PTH averages on the different pro tours are interesting to look at and compare to. You may not be trying to make a career out of golf but it's good to see what the best players do. Year in, year out, the leading player from 50–125 yards (45–114 metres) is somewhere around 15 feet PTH. That's the *leading* player. The average is a few feet higher, so hitting a wedge to 20 feet isn't too shabby at all. A wedge to 30 feet at Royal Melbourne, for example, can be an amazing shot given how firm the greens get. On other courses a wedge to 20 feet might be an ordinary shot if the greens are as soft as puddings.

Finally, it's important to build into your full-swing sessions time with these clubs. At the very least work on the three-quarter swing for each wedge and, with practice, it'll become a favourite shot. To up the ante, work on the three swings (half, three-quarter, full) and hit to different targets with each wedge. Some yardages will overlap. For example, the three-quarter pitching wedge might go the same as your full-swing gap wedge. This provides options on the course when the pin is at the front or back of a green or tucked in the corner, or when greens are hard or soft. Being able to control these shots consistently provides more freedom in other parts of your game knowing that the wedges can cover for you.

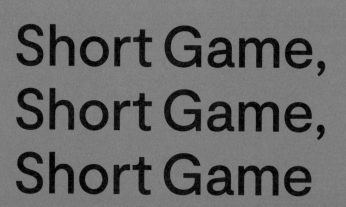

Short Game,
Short Game,
Short Game

In my early years on the European Tour I was fortunate enough to play with the late, great Severiano Ballesteros a couple of times. I've now come to truly appreciate what a genius he was. Normally I didn't pay much attention to playing partners, instead focusing on my own game. With Seve though, I couldn't help myself. One round in particular was at the Irish Open in 2001. His ball striking was awful, which wasn't surprising, as his full swing had disintegrated well before then. However, when faced with a shot requiring some creativity, his game sprung to life. Same for anything inside wedge distance of the hole. His imagination and touch on shorter shots was phenomenal. To the casual observer, if you saw him tee off each hole, breaking 80 would have been out of the question. But, at the end of the round, he signed for 72. There are great short games, and then there's the master — Seve.

The point being, players adept with the shorter clubs always have a chance of scoring well. Almost two-thirds of strokes taken in a round of golf are from wedge distance and in, mostly comprised of putts, with a mix of chips, pitches, bunker shots and wedges thrown in as well. It's no coincidence the names on leaderboards at the end of each week are usually the ones high up in scrambling stats. Sure, players on tour hit the ball well, but those that recover best around the greens are the contenders at week's end. This chapter is about chipping, pitching and bunker play.

Chipping

Much like the golf swing, there are differing views on chipping technique and various ways to do it well. As always, figure out what works best for you, but for me, a good set-up is the foundation and simplifies the rest. You can't go wrong with a narrow and slightly open stance, weight more on the left side, and hands a touch ahead of the ball. Simple. Ball position can vary but middle of the stance is just fine. From there, and after watching the best chippers in the world and experimenting myself, I've found two common elements to become good and a third to be great.

RHYTHM AND TEMPO

Like putting, distance in chipping is more important than line. With good distance control you'll rarely be more than a few paces away, unless there's quite a bit of slope and you've misread the break. With poor distance control, 20 feet short or long is common. Controlling distance requires solid contact, which comes from good rhythm and tempo. Tempos can vary in speed (as previously discussed), but the overall rhythm should be smooth. When golfers have a quick and jerky action, it's because their backswing is too short. To get the necessary distance they speed up on the through swing (I don't call it a downswing). For those that decelerate, their backswing is too long and they slow down to prevent hitting the ball too far. Both scenarios lead to chunks, skulls and miss-hits in general.

The transition from backswing to through swing is where most problems occur. Focus on making a smooth transition in relation to your tempo. If your tempo is quicker, continue the transition in the same fashion, and likewise for a slower tempo. Like putting, if your backswing is longer, your overall tempo will be slower. For a shorter backswing, the tempo will be faster. From there it's much easier to find the natural rhythm and tempo that suits you. A good rule of thumb is how far you take the club back is equal to how far the club follows through.

CONNECTION

The second part of good chipping is the connection between your arms, hands and lower body. I like to think of my hips (or trunk) dictating the motion, with everything else along for the ride. Some say the lower body should lead, but I've found golfers start using their knees too much, creating more problems. If your hips turn through correctly, your legs follow accordingly. Having an open stance at set-up and turning out the left foot helps to promote this turn too. I find a square stance/left foot restricts the hips on the shorter shots. With the hips leading the way there's a lovely smoothness to the motion. The hands and arms become an extension upon which the club is delivered to the ball.

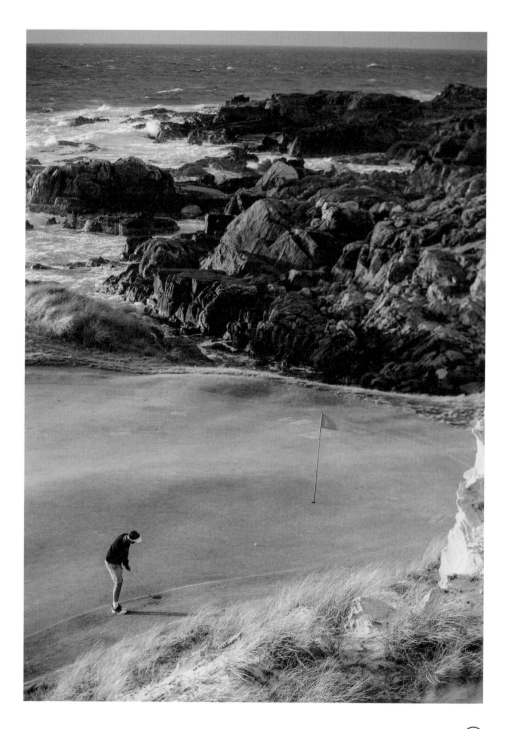

Drill

Get in your set-up position for a chip shot, but rather than a club in your hands, place a ball in your right hand and place your left hand behind your back. Make a backswing as usual, then turn through and release the ball in an underarm fashion to your target. Deliver the ball with the hips, arm and hand all working together – not the hand and arm separately doing the work. The goal is to have the right hand, arm and hips moving together so the ball is released slightly on the follow-through in a nice soft trajectory.

GREAT CHIPPING IS IN THE HANDS

The best chippers have great hands that caress the club for a lovely, soft touch. It looks like the ball is on a string. Lydia Ko has one of the best short games in the world and is an ideal player to watch in this regard. You can't create this touch if you are strangling the club because you lose the feel of the clubface. The greats are able to manipulate the clubface with their hands from difficult and tricky lies. Going back to Seve, his chip shot on the 72nd hole at Royal Lytham during the Open Championship in 1988 was one of the all-time great chip shots. After missing the green pin-high left, he needed to get up and down from an awkward lie to win. What followed is something definitely worth looking up on YouTube. With the ball nestled down in long grass and below his feet, he hit an exquisite chip that popped out, rolled a good 40 feet, gently kissed the lip of the cup before coming to rest 6 inches away. Good chippers can get the ball close from normal lies. Great ones do the same from tough lies under extreme pressure, making the difficult seem simple.

DIFFERING STYLES

There are two main styles of chipping. The first is an action that takes the angles out of the motion through less wrist hinge and with more body rotation. Steve Stricker is an exponent of this style. It can look like an extended putting motion from a chipping set-up. The other style is on the artistic side, with more softness and feel in the hands. These players tend to be wristier, Seve being the prime example. For people that struggle with chipping and tend to miss-hit a lot of shots, the Stricker method is the one I'd recommend. With fewer moving parts, fewer things can go wrong – and it's easier to find the low point of the chipping action with this method. Once comfortable, introduce the hands a little more for feel shots and see how you go. But again, find the style that feels most comfortable for you.

DIFFERENT TURF AND LIES

Playing off varying ground conditions – firmer and softer ground, for example – can give golfers the fits. In Melbourne, the ground can be rock hard around the greens, especially in summer, making solid contact difficult. Off firm, tight lies, the club can easily bounce off the ground resulting in thinned shots. To prevent this, use the leading edge more by standing taller and closer to the ball so the hands are higher. The toe of the club will feel on the ground rather than the heel. For some, in reality, the club will lay flat because quite a number of golfers have the toe slightly off the ground to begin with. By 'toeing down' the club, it helps the leading edge strike the ball first. It feels like you're 'pinching' the ball off the turf. Leaning your hands ahead of the ball more than usual is also a good idea.

From softer ground there's more room for error. The clubhead glides through easier so a regular set-up is fine. Soft, grainy grass can present problems though, and experimenting with shaft lean and ball position is something to play around with. Down grain is easier; into the grain is the trickier one. On these the leading edge wants to dig into the ground, since the grain opposes the direction you're swinging. My way of counteracting this is different to most, by choice because it works for me. I come into the ball slightly steeper to get to the back of the ball without any interference from the grain. It can look as though I'm 'stubbing' the shot because there's very little follow-through. It's high risk but I'm confident in this method. The more conventional way I'd recommend for most golfers is to play the shot with less shaft lean and a shallower angle of attack using the bounce of the club more rather than the leading edge. The key is to make sure you turn through the ball with little wrist hinge. Getting 'handsy' on these and not turning through the ball is where most problems occur.

Sloping lies require aligning yourself with the slope so you're able to swing with it (much like the full swing). Downhill chip shots prove more difficult because golfers don't widen their stance enough to be able to shift weight into their left side, creating the necessary stability to swing down with the slope. All it takes is some experimentation. Try different clubs too. It's not always the lob wedge or one of the wedges. Playing a bump and run with a less lofted club can be a much smarter play because miss-hits are better than with more lofted clubs.

Drill

Out of 10: Throw 10 balls in every direction around a green, ideally out on the course, but if not, around the practice green is fine. Play each ball as it lies for a variety of lies and stances.

Option 1: use the same club for each shot.

Option 2: use a club appropriate for each shot.

If you're able to putt each ball out, see how many you can get up and down out of 10. If not, how many can you get within a flagstick length of the hole. Keep score and repeat on the next green if you're on the course. On the practice green, switch holes and start again.

Find someone at your club with a renowned short game. Watch how they hit certain shots and pick their brains about how they do it. It never hurts to ask.

Lee Janzen, the two-time US Open champion, was (and still is) a member of Isleworth while I was there. On the short-game area one day I was watching him hit these lovely soft shots out of thick rough with what looked like an unusual hooking action. His feel was to lay the face open and take a long, rounded swing that came into the ball quite shallow. Usually out of thicker rough it's better to come in steeper, but his ball popped out high and soft every time. It looked like a bunker shot from soft sand with a very flat swing. I started experimenting with the shot and it came in handy on US courses because they love growing rough right up to the green's edge. Lee has an incredible short game and if you're able to watch him on the Champions Tour take note of his soft hands. It looks like he can get the ball up and down from anywhere – and usually he does.

I rarely speak of equipment, but having the right amount of bounce on your wedges can help with playing off different turf depending on your tendencies. For example, if you have a habit of chunking chip shots, more bounce can help by the club not digging as much at impact. Conversely, if you thin shots more often than not, less bounce can help the club dig into the ground more through the shot. We all have no hesitation in getting fitted for a driver, but wedges are just as important. I've always had a soft spot for the wedges Bob Vokey builds for Titleist. They come in a variety of grinds that look and feel fantastic. Plus, he's one of the nicest blokes you could hope to meet. The same goes for Ping and the clubs they produce. I've used their woods, irons and putters throughout my entire career. They go above and beyond to make sure the equipment is spot-on for their players.

Finally, with chipping don't be afraid to use different clubs to see which one is right for the shot. Earlier on I mentioned the 'Five clubs to one target' drill (page 29). Use the same action with different clubs and you'll quickly get an idea which is the correct club for the shot.

Pitching

Pitching is a slightly longer version of the chipping action and the best way to become good at this area of the game is practice, plain and simple. The hardest part is distance control. Getting a feel for how far the ball flies – and how it reacts when it lands – takes repetition. The set-up and motion are the same as chipping. We're just making a longer backswing, and because of this, a little more wrist hinge is involved. The further we take the club back, the more the hands come into it. On the through swing, still feel the hips, arms, and hands working together through the shot, rather than just the arms and hands. Being handsy makes distance control tough, unless you have great feel. Jason Day is an ideal player to observe. He has almost no wrist hinge on his backswing and follow-through for chipping and pitching, instead using his trunk to rotate back and through. It can look wooden, but the results speak for themselves, as he's one of the best in the game around the greens.

Drill

Pick a shot of, say, 55 yards (50 metres) and use all your different wedges to pitch the ball and finish pin high. In my case, I'd use the 60-, 54- and 46-degree wedges. With the same action, vary the length of the backswing for each club to get the desired result distance-wise. Observe the different trajectories and how far the ball rolls out when it lands.

'Jason Day is an ideal player to observe. He has almost no wrist hinge on his backswing and follow-through for chipping and pitching, instead using his trunk to rotate back and through.'

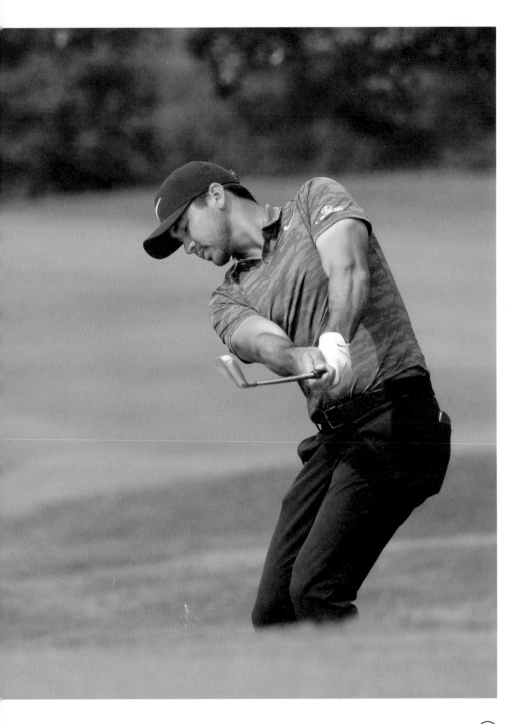

Short Game, Short Game, Short Game

Bunkers

Watching a great bunker player is mesmerising. The sound the club makes as it thumps into the sand is very different to the sound an average bunker player makes. Back in the day Norman Von Nida had no equal from bunkers and I understand he taught Gary Player everything he knows about playing from the sand. Seve Ballesteros, Peter 'Chook' Fowler and Tony Johnstone are some of the best I've ever seen, along with Brett Rumford in recent years. I played with Tony in Spain on the European Tour years ago, where he had three bunker shots during the round. He holed one, lipped out another and left the third 2 feet away. Yeah, not bad.

Again, opinions vary as to the correct method, but to start, here are some fundamentals I recommend for a stock bunker shot off a flat lie in decent sand. Like chipping, the set-up is important. Widen the stance, aim the feet slightly left of target, lean your weight into the left side (keep it there throughout the swing) and open up the clubface. Hinge your wrists on the backswing more than usual, then accelerate through the ball striking the sand a few inches or so behind it and follow through. I see lots of players on tour using a square stance, which is fine. See what works for you.

Gary Player has a great video where he talks about setting the wrists early on the backswing, then 'lighting the match' on the through swing, which helps create speed through the ball by unhinging the wrists on the follow-through. Too many golfers either try and lift the ball out or decelerate and don't follow through in fear of hitting it too far. Both lead to either fat or thinned shots. By opening the clubface and hitting down through the ball with speed, the bounce on the sole of the sand wedge is exposed to the sand and does the work for you.

As is the case with all shots, the lie dictates everything in bunkers. Once we've assessed that, adapt accordingly. For example, is the ball sunk down in the sand? Or is it perched cleanly on top? If it's sitting down, the ball won't have as much spin when it lands. From good, clean lies more spin can be created. There are numerous factors to consider because every situation is different, and a lot can be determined as we dig our feet in. The following are some guidelines to follow.

SOFT SAND

Softer sand tends to have a fine, powdery look and feels heavier underfoot. Deep rake marks near the ball from the bunker machine or rake are a giveaway too. The clubhead wants to dig in soft sand, so it's important to use the bounce by opening up the clubface. It's there for a reason – to bounce off the sand and explode the ball out. With a square clubface, the leading edge takes over, digging in behind the ball resulting in heavy, fat shots. The same goes for hitting down too steeply into the ball. From softer sand, a shallower swing allows the club to move through the sand more easily. Too steep and it's tough going. For a higher trajectory, open the face way up, aim further left and make a fuller, harder swing. But remember, don't try and lift the ball out. Keep your weight on the left side, swing through the ball and it will come out high and soft. The hard part is trusting this, but that's more about being committed.

HARD SAND

A baked, crusty appearance and lighter feel walking into a bunker usually means a firmer lie. On these occasions we don't want to use the bounce as much because it skims the clubhead off the sand resulting in bladed shots. By squaring up the clubface more, the leading edge can dig in first and get under the ball effectively. A steeper angle of attack from more wrist hinge on the backswing helps from firmer lies too. A shallower swing can lead to the club bouncing off the sand. Typically, you won't need as long a backswing because the clubhead doesn't interact with the sand as much, so the ball comes out a little quicker. Play from wet sand in the same fashion. Rain compacts the sand making it firmer, thus using the leading edge is necessary.

SLOPED LIES

Like all sloped lies, we want to align our body to the slope and swing with it. Widen your stance and build a base by digging the feet in. This allows you to move your weight around and stay balanced. Downhill bunker shots are the most difficult because golfers try and lift the ball out rather than trusting the loft on the clubface. Shift extra weight into your left side to help swing down with the slope and through the ball. Open the clubface more if there's a high lip to carry, and keep all the other principles the same. The ball will fly lower and release more, so keep this in mind. The opposite is true for uphill lies. The ball flies higher and lands softer, and it's mostly all carry to the target. When the ball is below the feet, aim further left and exaggerate your knee bend at set-up to help get down and under the ball. Hinging the wrists more vertically on the backswing helps too. When the ball's above our feet, the club wants to dig into the sand resulting in fat shots. To counteract this, feel a more rounded swing for a shallower angle of attack into the sand. Aim further right as the ball goes left off these lies. For all the above shots, staying balanced throughout the swing is vital.

PLUGGED LIES

How severely a ball is plugged determines our expectations. Sometimes just getting the ball on the green is a victory. Other times it's realistic to get the ball close. For all bunker shots we want to follow through, bar this one. All our energy is going down into the sand behind the ball to extract it, so the follow-through doesn't matter. We're trying to dig the ball out by attacking it from a steep angle. To do this, square the clubface up and lean heavily into the left leg. An image I use on extreme plugged lies is to chop wood. It encourages a very sharp downward angle to get under the ball. How badly it's plugged determines how steep you attack it. The ball comes out with no spin and may squirt right a little, so allow for both. Getting the ball close is a real possibility if it's not too deep and there's plenty of green to work with, or a plugged lie in an upslope usually isn't too bad either if it's not too deep. Using a gap wedge or lower lofted wedge is also an option too.

For all bunker shots, how much sand to take behind the ball varies depending on the sand's texture and the lie.

Drill

Line in the sand: Place 10 balls in a row and draw a line in the sand behind each one where you want the club to enter. By hitting the line behind each ball, you'll quickly get a feel for how much sand is too much or too little depending on the lie.

LONG BUNKER SHOTS

These shots pose problems for many golfers but, like chipping, a good solution is to change clubs depending on the shot. For example, on a 27-yard (25-metre) bunker shot with plenty of green to work with, you don't have to use the lob wedge. In fact, I'm against it (unless the lip is very high). Instead, try a gap wedge, pitching wedge, even a 9-iron. You'll be amazed how much easier these clubs are for longer bunker shots. Keep the set-up, open clubface and action the same, just remember that a 27-yard (25-metre) bunker shot with a pitching wedge is like a 11-yard (10-metre) bunker shot with a lob wedge. You don't have to swing harder – the club will do the work. The ball comes out lower, with less spin and releases further. It just takes practice.

Poor shots with less-lofted clubs are better than with higher-lofted ones. Think about it. A thinned lob wedge with a full-blooded swing is going way over the green. A thinned pitching wedge bunker shot with a shorter swing will only go 20 or 30 feet past the target. Same goes for chunking both. A chunked pitching wedge will get much closer to the hole than a chunked lob wedge.

SHORT-SIDED BUNKER SHOTS

For normal bunker shots I use what I call a U-shape swing (if you look at the swing's shape from side on). A U-shape swing is like a normal swing but with a little more wrist hinge on the backswing and follow through. On short-sided bunker shots where I need to get the ball up sharply and stopping quickly, I go for a V-shape swing. For a V-shape swing, hinge the wrists sharply up on the backswing and on the through swing. From the side it looks like a V-shape. It requires clubface awareness and a deft touch. If your handicap's in double figures I'd take the safer option and play past the pin. However, if you fancy your chances give it a go. But practise it first!

Drill

Three-iron bunker shots: This sounds hard and it is. You need a lot of hand manipulation and a unique set-up to hit these from a greenside bunker. Widen your stance to the extreme so your hands are as low as possible. Hinge the club sharply up on the way back and also on the way through. If you're able to get a few out and on the green, bravo. If not, no worries, it's not easy, and using a 3-iron is more for elite players. For everyone else start with a 7-iron instead, and if successful, then try a 5-iron. In any case when you go back to the sand wedge after using the 3-, 5- or 7-iron, the sand wedge becomes a piece of cake. This drill is part of my skill work in a practice session.

I heard Seve used to do this as a youngster because he only had a 3-iron growing up. Figuring out different shots with it became second nature and one of the main reasons he was a short-game genius. Throughout Seve's career the highest loft he ever used was a 56-degree sand wedge because he didn't feel the need for a 60-degree.

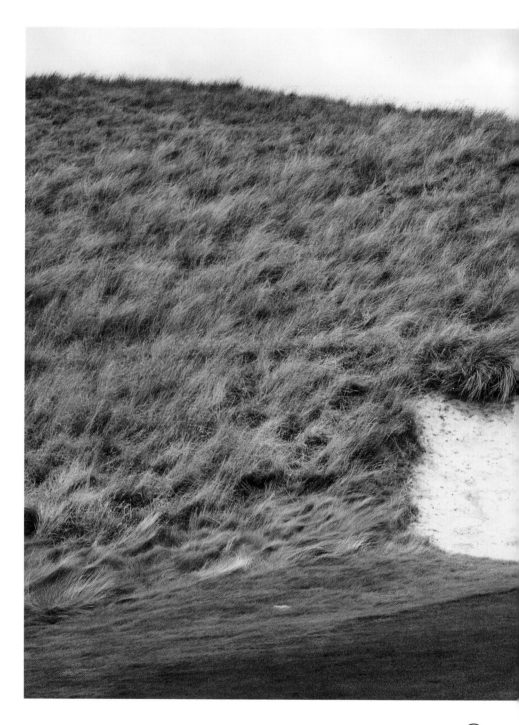

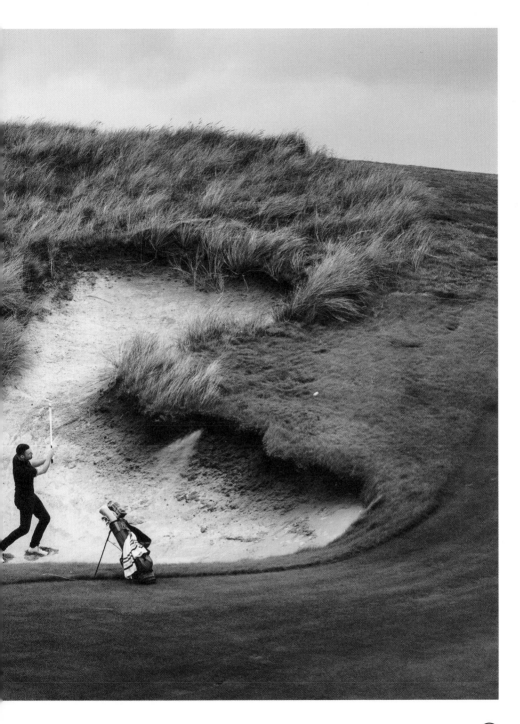

Short Game, Short Game, Short Game

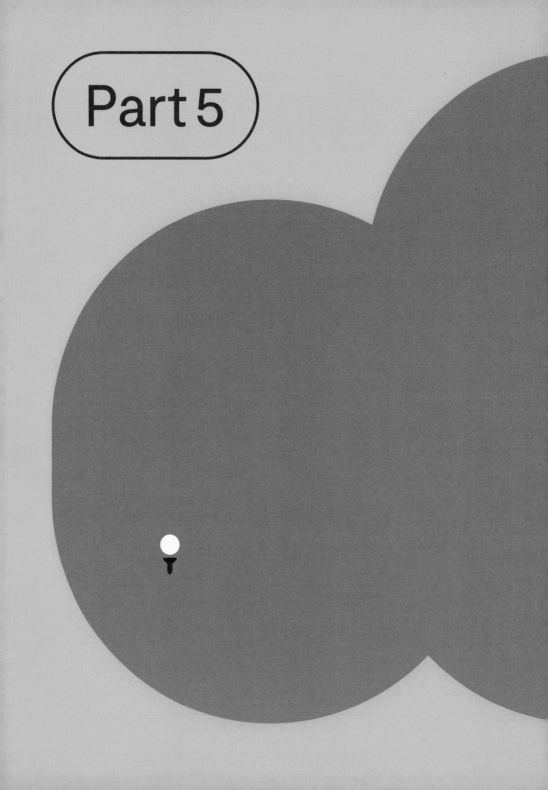

Part 5

A Game Like No Other

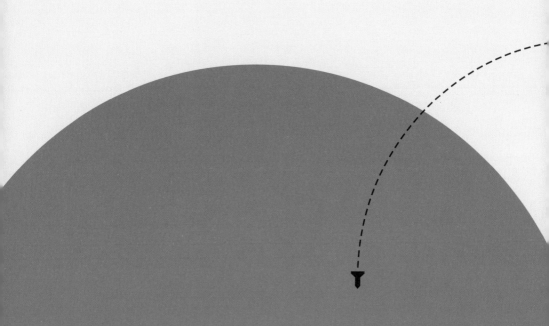

Being a Rookie

For aspiring pros looking to make a career from the game, this chapter is for you. For everyone else, it's an insight into the trials and tribulations of life on tour.

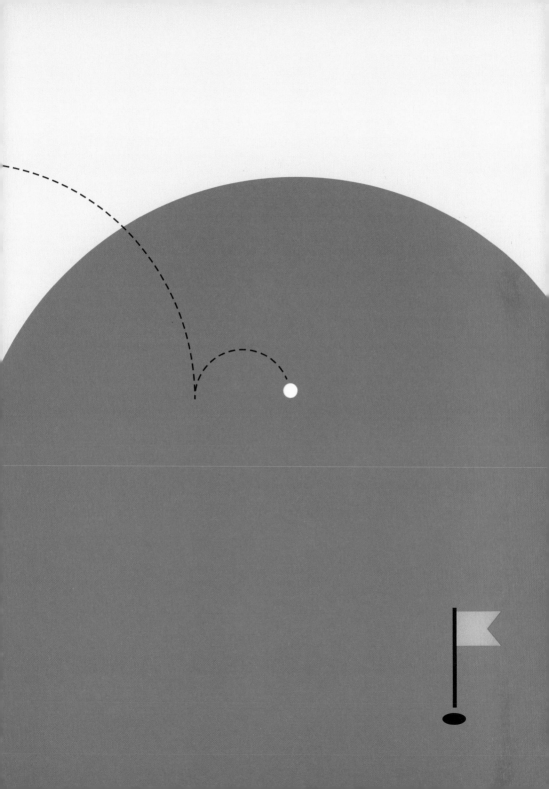

The first year on any tour is the hardest. There are numerous obstacles to overcome, mostly figured out simply by going through the experience. Off the course, there's the travel factor – airports, hotels, delays, lost luggage, eating out, different time zones, jetlag – the list goes on. Golf-wise, it's fitting in time to practise, figuring out courses you've never seen, hiring a good caddy, dealing with agents, manufacturing companies and their reps, working out in the gym and so on. A week on tour is literally like a travelling circus.

My rookie season in Europe was an incredible eye-opener and I'm forever thankful to Paul Norris, a businessman from Brisbane, Queensland. I got my card at the 1998 European Tour Qualifying School in the south of Spain and straight after, my wife, Alana, and I flew back to play a couple of events on the Aussie circuit, including the Coolum Classic on Queensland's Sunshine Coast. At that stage Coolum was a pro-am format (like the Dunhill Links Championship in Scotland) and over the first three days, Paul, a fellow lefty, was my partner. We hit it off straight away and at the traditional Friday Cut Party, he asked how Alana and I were going to cope the following year in Europe with all the costs. I remember saying, 'I'm not sure but we'll figure it out.' To which he replied, 'How about I pay your expenses for the year in return for a percentage of prize money until they're paid off. After that I'll reduce the percentage, and if you don't make enough to cover expenses, that's okay.' Alana and I couldn't believe it. Paul wasn't offering the deal to make money. It was to help relieve the initial financial stress we were in for, an amazing gesture. It freed me up to just play golf, and we later learned he'd done the same for a few other players. What a guy!

' In searing humidity,
a lasting memory was the
local monkeys climbing
out of overhanging trees
down into our golf carts
during the pro-am pilfering
whatever they could –
food, wallets, phones. I'd
never seen anything like it.'

My first event for the 1999 season was, funnily enough, in my home town of Perth, Australia. An odd place to start, given it's the European Tour, but back then the Heineken Classic, at the Vines Golf Club, was a co-sanctioned event with the PGA Tour of Australasia. I finished T36, not bad but not great either. The week after was another co-sanctioned event, this time with the Asian Tour, in Kuala Lumpur at the Saujana Country Club. In searing humidity, a lasting memory was the local monkeys climbing out of overhanging trees down into our golf carts during the pro-am pilfering whatever they could — food, wallets, phones. I'd never seen anything like it. Saujana was a tough course requiring accurate ball striking. Fortunately, that was a strength of mine as the T11 finish showed. After that my ranking from Q-School didn't get me in another tournament until six weeks later, the Madeira Islands Open off the coast of Portugal.

There's a saying on tour, 'You only play Madeira once', and we learned why later. To get there, Alana and I flew from Perth to Singapore to London to Lisbon to Madeira — all up a 36-hour trip. Not much fun in the back of the plane, let me tell you. The Madeira airport, at the time, had one of the shortest runways in the world perched on the side of a mountain, and, apparently, the pilots only had a small area in which to touch down the plane to be able to stop in time. Another problem was high winds frequented the area, so landing was extremely difficult. Overshooting the mark meant dropping off the end of the runway and down the mountain — not ideal really. Before the runway was a cliff face so, understandably, they tended to be long rather than short. Too long and they'd pull the plane up quickly to circle back and try again. We didn't know all this (thankfully) and touched down first try. After the plane slowed down, people began clapping, which was baffling to us. The person in the next seat explained it usually took two or three tries to successfully land. Being so tired from the long journey it didn't register; we just wanted to find our accommodation and sleep. The following morning, the bus ride from the hotel to the course was back up the mountain past the airport. Driving by, Alana and I looked at each other and thought, 'We landed on that?' I was so glad we didn't know because Alana is not a good flyer. To this day if we're on a plane for a golf-related trip, she holds up her wine glass (because that always helps calm the nerves) and gives me a dirty look. Poor love.

Over the next six months we visited Portugal, Spain, France, England, Germany, Morocco, Ireland, Scotland, the Netherlands, Sweden and Switzerland, with multiple trips back to a few of those in between. Culture shock was an understatement. It sounds like the greatest trip ever, but when your living relies on how you perform on a golf course, the allure wears off pretty quick. However, amongst all that, we rented an apartment with Jarrod and Danielle Moseley in Virginia Water, a quaint village in Surrey about 40 minutes from Heathrow airport near London. Jarrod won the Heineken event in Perth earlier in the year and was fully exempt on tour, so we thought to cut costs sharing the rent was a good solution.

I learned invaluable lessons that first year, some the hard way, some through simply asking questions. As a rule, seasoned players on tour are quite willing to share information if asked, and as I came to realise, that's all you have to do – ask. Some players aren't so inclined, which is understandable since we're all out there with the same goal. Peter Senior and Wayne Riley were two players very gracious to Alana and me, sharing tips on where to eat, places to stay and the like. Bits of information like this go a long way for a rookie. These small details add up and every piece of advice is greatly appreciated.

Through all this Alana had been caddying. After making the first five cuts, we experimented with having a different caddy on the bag for a few events. Upon which I proceeded to miss the next three cuts in a row. We knew there'd come a time when I'd need a full-time professional caddy, but three straight missed cuts put an end to that idea right away (until Wilbur came along the following year). Alana was straight back on the bag for a sixth-place finish in Morocco the next week. As it happened, both of us came down with food poisoning during the tournament – another joy of international travel. The golf bag was stocked with rolls of toilet paper as we took turns running off into the bushes when the urge struck.

The rest of the year was up and down, until finally I secured my card for the following season at the Omega European Masters in Crans-sur-Sierre, Switzerland, with a T9 finish. After closing with a 3-under-par 68, Alana and I hugged in pure relief knowing we'd wrapped up my playing rights for the following year. In all I made 12 of 18 cuts with two top 10s and seven top-25 finishes to finish 108th on the Order of Merit. At the end of each year, the top 115 kept their cards, so for my first year, it felt like a very successful season.

It was my first time playing every golf course we visited, bar the Vines in Perth. Competing at a high level on a course you've never seen is not easy. Experience is a valuable tool because you know which pins you can and can't go at, areas to avoid, how greens break and so on. One thing I learned was to walk the course the first time rather than play it. This way, my initial look was unbiased. By playing it first, my interpretation of a hole could be dictated by how I played that day. Plus, it didn't give me a chance to see certain parts of the course. For example, if I drove it down the right on a hole, I didn't see the left side and perhaps there was vital information over there. By walking a course first, you see more of its intricacies that go unnoticed otherwise. Now, if you only get one chance to see a course beforehand then, yes, play it. It's important to get a feel for how far the ball is flying, rolling out on the fairways, reacting on the greens and so forth.

My first year in Europe was a huge challenge. Everything was magnified because each week there was a different language and culture to adapt to as well as the golf. When I first started playing in the US, the transition was easier. Every week you're in the same country. There's always a Starbucks, Chipotle and Whole Foods, no matter where you are. They were my go-to places for coffee, a quick easy meal and a health-food store to get the week's supplies. Visit any of these while a tour event's in town and trust me, there'll be plenty of pros in each one. In some European cities, restaurants don't open until 9 pm, and finding a convenience store trading on a Sunday? Impossible. But you adapt quickly and learn much more about yourself in these situations. It's why I recommend young pros try the European Tour before the PGA Tour. Being flexible and adaptable is a must in this game and the European Tour is the ultimate test for both.

I didn't really have a rookie year in the US because initially I was top 50 in the world rankings and was still playing the European Tour. This ranking enabled me to start making trips across the pond to play the majors, World Golf Championship events and several tournaments on invites. I did this for a couple of years and, given how I was playing, felt very comfortable going back and forth. The toughest part was the amount of travel involved. I would have loved to continue playing both tours, but it wasn't feasible as Alana and I had a baby daughter with another on the way. We needed stability rather than constant toing and froing.

My first full year on the PGA Tour was 2007 and I was already well accustomed to playing there, so the move was much smoother. Looking back, the 1999 season in Europe was the most important year. I learned more about my game than any other year on tour. Navigating it successfully instilled the confidence and the belief I was good enough to play at the highest level. Once Wilbur was on my bag early the next season, every year that followed was a steady climb up the ladder. The initial 'Do I belong out here?' question was quickly put to rest. What I realised was, if you are good enough to get on tour, you have the game to stay there.

The only thing I'd do differently would be to play more practice rounds with the top players and ask more questions on and off the course. It's part of the reason I've started mentoring golfers now. Not that I'm an expert, but I can provide insights and knowledge from my experience that may be useful with their journey. The learning curve for young pros can be quicker by talking and playing with past and present players rather than trying to figure things out all by themselves.

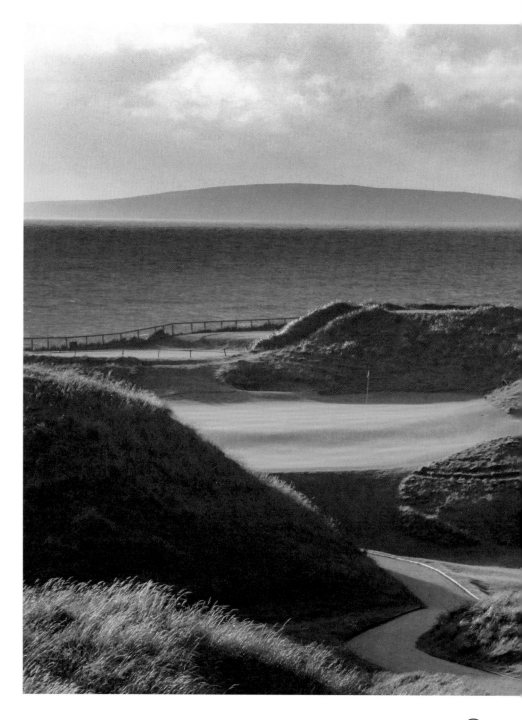

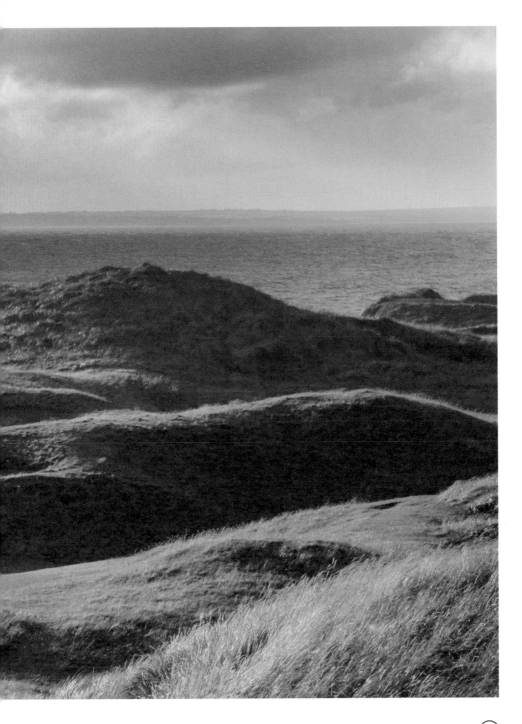

Caddying: An Insider's Take

BY JAMES 'WILBUR' WILLIAMS

In *Tour Mentality*, I asked Alana to write a chapter because she's seen my entire journey in pro golf. This time, I thought I'd get my old caddy, Wilbur, to give you his take on one of the oldest pastimes in the game.

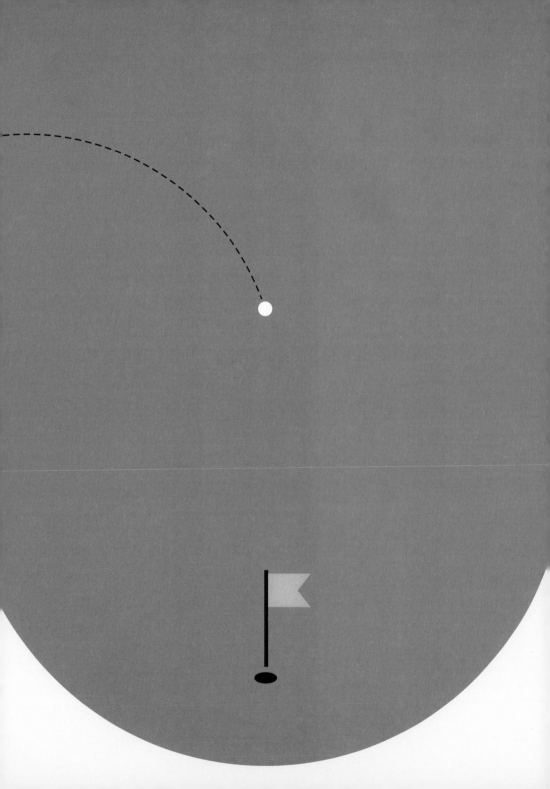

My first tournament as a professional caddy was the Catalan Open, outside Barcelona, in March 1996. A friend of mine, Gary, caddied for DJ Russell on the European Tour, and after chatting about his job one day, I somehow found myself on a plane to Spain, with hardly any money, no bag arranged and shitting myself. Once we landed, Gary spoke to a few other caddies and players, and before I knew it Liam White, an English tour pro with a fantastic pedigree, came over and said, 'I'm looking for a caddy, are you fixed?'

I had myself a bag.

At the time I had no idea what to do, where to go, what to organise, what time to be where – the list seemed endless. With no mobile phone in those days, it was just pure verbal communication. Liam was a great first boss. I carried the bag, tried not to put him off, kept out of his way, shagged practice balls, replaced divots (lots of them), fetched coffee, watched, listened and asked questions when I thought it was safe to do so. Needless to say, asking or saying something at the wrong time has a player's head coming off thick and fast. But you learn and learn quickly.

Being 21 years old, my first three years blurred into one massive holiday. I loved caddying, and travelling and didn't mind staying in one-star hotels for a week, or even on the odd carpet floor. Having a few drinks at night got you through the weeks where crappy hotels were non-negotiable. Money came in and went out, and sometimes stayed out.

Missed cuts – it's basic really. If your player makes the cut, you earn a percentage of their winnings. Miss the cut, and it's a weekend off or you're on the range practising. The latter means spending more cash while earning no extra. Adjusting your mind to accept this took a few years to sink in, but eventually it did.

Everything changed at a tournament in Morocco '98. I was grinding from week to week, learning and gaining experience as a rookie amongst caddy 'lifers' of the tour. At a hotel bar one evening I started chatting to a lifer named Seagull (every caddy has a nickname), who'd been on tour 25 years and worked for players such as Eduardo Romero, Mark McNulty and at one point a very young Nick Faldo, among many others. At the time Tiger Woods was tightening his grip on the world's golfing scene and the conversation with Seagull centred around Tiger. Tournament purses were going up quickly and with caddies getting 10 per cent of a player's cheque for a win (that's all we thought about), he said if he was my age, young, single and keen, he'd make a career at caddying. I didn't realise you could have a career; I thought caddying would never last. From that conversation on I never looked back. I reined things in, knuckled down, asked loads of questions of the players I worked for, and grew as a person and as a caddy.

Caddy lessons – keep up, shut up (when it's needed) and show up early because if you're not early you're late. This will never change.

The first time I saw Nick was at the 2000 Spanish Open in Girona while working for Gary Evans. Also in our group was the late Gordon Brand Jnr. All I thought was, 'Who is Nick O'Hern and OMG he's left-handed!' I clearly remember on the first green Nick had 30 feet, rolled it in dead centre, perfect pace. Through 7 holes he was 3 under then holed a 6-iron from the fairway on the 8th. Nice 2, 5 under through 8. At the end Nick was tied for the lead after the first round with 'The Fish' (filling in for Alana) on the bag. What stood out was he was totally in control of what he was doing, not being greedy, just quietly going about his business and playing golf.

Fast-forward two weeks to the Benson & Hedges tournament at the Belfry in the middle of England and I'd parted ways with Gary after he MC'd (that's caddy talk for 'missed the cut'). It happens, caddies get sacked or sack players. I told The Fish I was looking and before I knew it, had a one-round trial with Nick during the last round of the B&H – how good! Nick's wife had caddied his first year and after securing full playing rights for the following season, she wanted out, so it was great timing. Knowing what I knew from seeing him play in Spain, I was really excited that Sunday. The usual routine was, I got a time to meet Nick in the locker room and was there 45 minutes early to get everything ready, only to be greeted by him 15 minutes earlier than expected. Little did I know then, Nick would arrive early for the next 12 f#%king years!

When you first caddy for anyone, the first time on the course, you just let them play. Do nothing except get the yardage and wind right, step back, watch and make notes discreetly. I remember asking for Nick's yardages (how far he hit everything) to have a starting point, however, he was quick to say, 'I'll do everything today, just do the yardage and get the wind right.' Perfect, no problems.

The hardest thing that day was standing on the left-hand side of the ball with the bag. Nick was the only left-handed golfer I'd ever worked for, and walking down the 1st hole, I put the bag on the right-hand side and got the yardage ... 0 for 1 ... then picked it up and moved it to the left. Nick hit his second shot just through the green but only 20 feet from the flag. Again, I put the bag down and realise I'm standing there looking at his arse. That's 0 for 2. It did my head in – lol! By the end we'd had a fun day and he'd played well. We were off and running. As I worked more and more with Nick, he naturally opened up and I could see his logic, path and process in what he was doing. He always said it's part of the process.

Nick hit every shot in the book, and had a touch of the old school, knocking down every club in his bag. A pure feel player. It could be flat calm or blowing 40 km/h and his distance control was ridiculously on point. This is something you always look for in a player. Under the cosh (gun), hitting your numbers always gives you a better chance of holing that putt to make the cut, force a playoff or win the trophy. Add in being a putting wizard, and all of a sudden, you had two serious moving parts to becoming a world-class golfer. I've been spoilt on the greens while working for Nick, watching him consistently hole it from everywhere, week in, week out. At one point, I might have shaken my head in disgust when he missed one from 40 feet – lol! He saw the short game as fun and a challenge instead of thinking, 'Shit, I best get this up and down', like others may think. The harder the shot the easier he made it – ridiculous! His short game was easily in the top 10 on the European Tour and continued the same across the pond on the PGA Tour.

Back in 2000 big hitters were 290 yards (265 metres) max off the tee, the majority of the field about 275. Nick averaged 260, not bad but if anything, short. But guess what, he split the fairway every time, and if under any kind of pressure, would tee it down, aim right and bunt driver about 245 yards (224 metres) low and with a 10-yard (9-metre) fade every single time without fail. It didn't matter what he had to hit in, it would be pin high or thereabouts, and with that putting stroke – watch out!

He was an absolute pleasure to work for He gave you confidence – and gave you stick and shit as and when you needed it. In good times and the not so good, Nick never changed, 100 per cent professional from the moment he put his shoes on in the locker room. He knew exactly what he was doing. His practice routines rarely changed although if extra was required in areas of his game, he got it done and never wasted time at the course or on the range. This is not to be underrated: at any tournament there are 20 to 30 players each day every week spending too much time at the course and over-practising. It's a fine line, but look at the results, look at the longevity of the world's best and do you see them up there 12 hours a day? Exactly.

'What makes a good caddy?' I've been asked this a load of times and there's no one answer, there's no secret. It comes from within, but a few traits you need are being able to deal with adversity, personalities, egos. You have to be a best mate, a cheerleader, a punching bag, a shrink, a sounding board, thick-skinned, competitive, reliable, flexible and committed to the cause. You have to not mind long hours, long flights and outlaying thousands of pounds/dollars to get to work. If you can handle all those, give it a go – when the bag is on your shoulder all the above disappears.

There are plenty of caddies on both the PGA and European Tours who haven't had the right break, or haven't made it happen for themselves. But in my eyes the best caddies consistently pop up and win tournaments with players who are not yet proven, or players who have gone missing for some years. These caddies ride a wave of fortune then have the foresight to see when the drive or passion leaves their golfer. They recognise their efforts are not appreciated and go off to work for someone else. And guess what? Yep, they show up with another player and win!

When you start working for someone who just got their card from tour school, or get an opportunity to work for an established player who's a big name, don't ever forget you didn't get them to where they are today. They got themselves there.

Confidence is the best thing you can give a golfer, whether it's someone in their first year on tour or their 10th. The only difference between them is the rookie doesn't have scar tissue (nothing tour-related anyway). The established player has seen, written and starred in their own disasters, but if you can get them to believe in themselves again, there's a good chance they'll push through the pain and onto greater things. The rookie has no real expectations, just big dreams. All this is surrounded by hard work, sacrifice and dedication with zero guarantee. However, if the belief is there, it more often comes true.

It's well documented now that caddies can earn a ridiculous amount of money for 22 to 30 weeks' work a year. Look at the top 10 Race to Dubai/FedEx Cup players and you do the maths. My motto is if you work hard at the right things, good things happen. For some caddies it happens quickly and continues to happen, others have a roller-coaster career. I count myself extremely lucky to have worked for some of the best golfers on the European and PGA Tours. I had some brilliant bosses and experienced luxuries I still can't believe to this day. It's all down to them and what they achieved. I just happened to have a ringside seat throughout all the highs and lows of this incredible game.

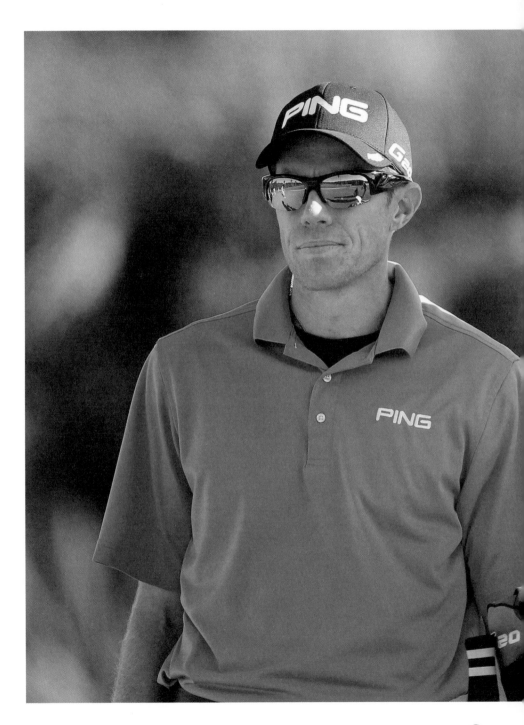

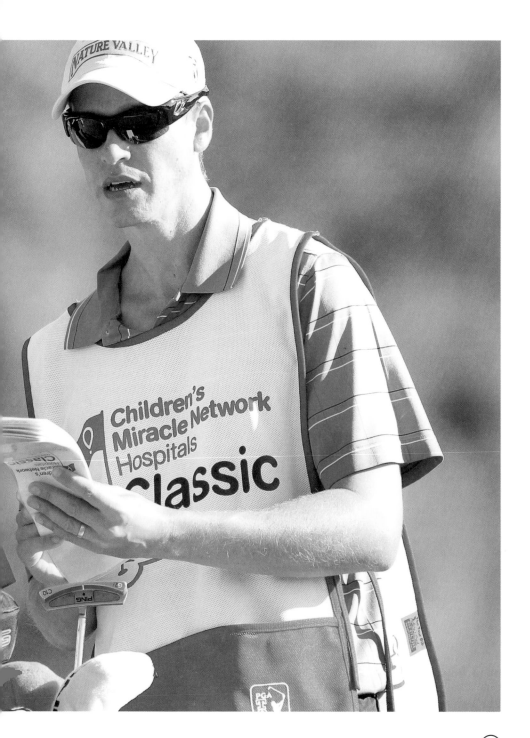

Caddying: An Insider's Take

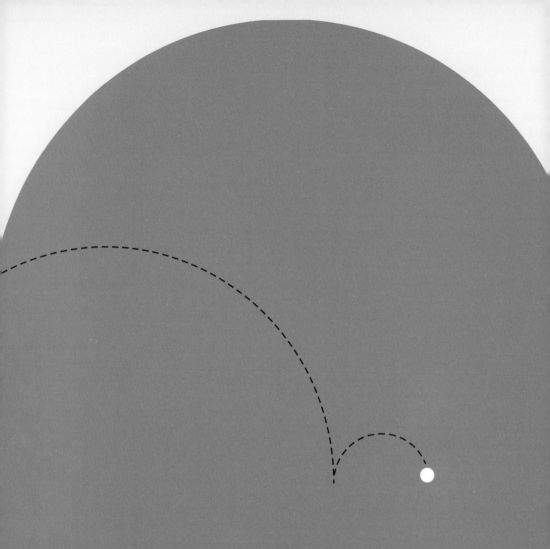

Become Your
Own Coach

Many years ago, my coach Neil Simpson said to me, 'I'm not your coach. I'm just someone who offers suggestions about your game. It's your choice whether you take them on board or not.' I was a little baffled by his comment, but over time it began to make sense. I had to trust my game implicitly because the only person who controlled my destiny on the course was me. If I faced a tough tee shot on the last hole of a tournament, I needed complete belief in what I was doing. Any doubt about my swing or mindset would be reflected in the result. Neil couldn't help right then. To some extent my caddy could, but I was the one hitting the shot and the buck stopped with me. It's why I love the game. Team sports were fun, but what always bugged me was I could play well, yet still lose. Whereas the 'it's all up to me' nature of golf is what initially drew me in. Having said that, playing in the Presidents Cup a couple of times reminded me how much fun having teammates can be!

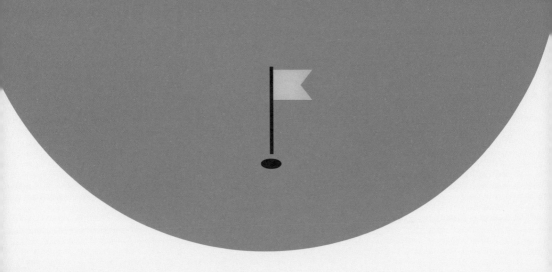

As you've read, scoring well is about being flexible, adapting to situations and figuring out what works for you. This last piece is different for everyone. What works for some may not work for others. My goal with this book is to provide suggestions for most scenarios you'll face on the course. (I say most because something new always pops up.) Now, it's up to you to choose what to incorporate into your game, experiment with and eventually *own*. How do you know what to take in and what to discard? To start, find someone who's a good sounding board to bounce ideas off, such as the local PGA pro at your club. Listening to golfers with higher handicaps generally isn't the wisest choice. Pros are trained in golf. Amateurs, well, they have day jobs for a reason.

Then it's trial and error to see what fits you best. When I took a lesson off Neil, he might suggest four or five different things. Internally I was saying, 'No I don't like that. Yes, I'll try that' and so on. Eventually I figured out he was saying the same thing, just in different ways. I had to connect with one of these in my own way, then go off and work on it so it became part of my game. Neil told me later his goal was to get me to a point where I didn't need him to fix things if I was away at a tournament. That's the sign of a great coach.

He found it quite amusing watching players at tournaments surrounded by their 'team' on the range. Everyone seemed to have an opinion and it looked sometimes as though the player ended up more confused at the end than when they started. In his typical dry way Neil used to say, 'If you're still working on your swing during a tournament, it's probably not going to be a good week.' He was spot-on as usual, for my best weeks were when I did little work on my swing, instead just focusing on what was required for that particular course.

Neil's definitely one of a kind and I'm forever thankful for his 'suggestions' over the years. Recently, while in Covid lockdown, I did an online course with Pareto People here in Melbourne called 'Coaching as a Leadership Style'. It was fascinating learning what coaching really is. It's actually not about telling someone what to do, but rather helping them find their own solutions through listening and asking questions. I'm now drawing on all my years of experience in the game and working with Pareto and their clients a few times a year with their development programs. Neil was an incredible coach in this regard, and his influence shaped my career. I still need help from time to time, but with his guidance, in a way I've become my own coach.

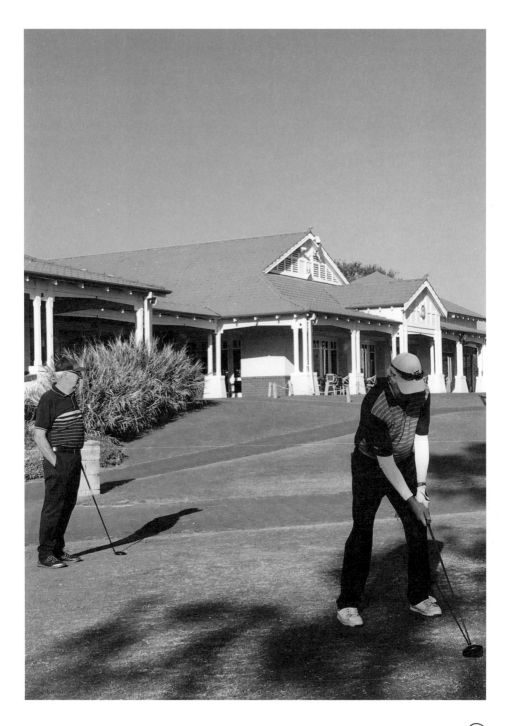

For the
Love of
the Game

I read a piece from a book a while ago by the late great Peter Thomson saying he'd gone full circle with his game. As a youngster, he hit the ball about 218 yards (200 metres) off the tee, scoring somewhere in the 80s. Then, at the height of his career he achieved amazing feats, including five Open Championships among many other highlights. In the latter stages of his playing days he'd come back to the 200-metre mark off the tee and scores in the 80s again, hence full circle. It's a beautiful way to look at the game. I'm not at this point yet, but in a way I see some similarities already. Not regarding length off the tee (although that will inevitably ensue), but more on how I started playing as a kid and now as a pro.

Growing up in Perth, the school bell at the end of each day signalled it was time to head off to the local public track, the Embleton Golf Course. My first set was made up of a 2-wood, a 3-, 5-, 7- and 9-iron, SW and putter. Every club was a different make and model with the shaft, grip and head of each bearing no resemblance to the others. Figuring out how each club flew was an art in itself. As my game progressed so too did the number of clubs in the bag, and I received my first matching full set at the age of 12. Golf was in my blood. Growing up, Dad taught me the fundamentals. The seed for making golf a career had been well and truly planted in my mid-teens after watching the Golden Bear, Jack Nicklaus, win The Masters in 1986. Initially I became a teaching pro (because I wasn't good enough to be a tour pro at that stage) before going on to play all the biggest tournaments in the world for many years. Toward the end, it became more a job than a passion and my love for the game began to wane as injuries interrupted my progress. Sitting in hotel rooms, I found myself not wanting to be there. I'd rather have been home with Alana and the kids.

Moving back to Australia recently has reinvigorated my passion for the game. I'm back to coaching and helping golfers again, coming full circle in that way as a pro. I love seeing the joy someone gets after helping them play better, and the joy has returned to my game too. I'm playing golf how I used to as a kid – in a creative, fun way with a half set. The irons are either odds or evens, to keep things interesting.

Playing with fewer clubs simplifies – yes, simplifies – the game. I'm never in between clubs because with fewer choices the right club is more obvious and the art of playing clearer. Pin high is all that matters, and the yardage almost becomes irrelevant. Give it a try sometime. Perhaps start with 10 clubs. Take out a few you rarely use. Then drop another and another. After a while you'll get a feel for which are the most versatile. It's liberating in a way to free yourself of all these options. Keeping things simple is how we play our best golf. Plus, golf's a walking game and it's much easier to carry a half set!

If you feel like you still need the yardage, by all means pull the laser out to get the distance, but after a while it will become an unnecessary gadget. Like ball washers, or scorecard holders. ☺ Your other senses will take over and the instincts for the right club and the right shot will continually develop. You'll become a golf-course player, someone who writes down their lowest score possible each time out ... and therein lies the art of playing golf.

Cheers,
Nick

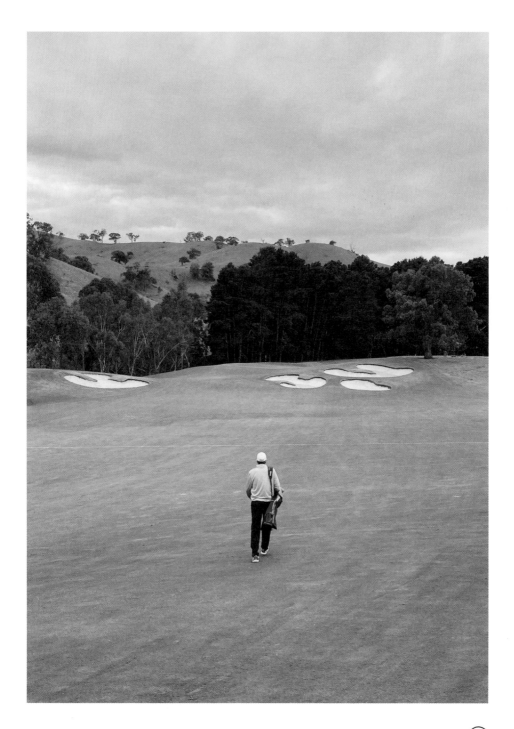

For the Love of the Game

About the author

Nick O'Hern is a highly respected pro golfer who was based in the US for most of his career and has only recently returned to Australia. He spent two decades playing professional golf at the highest level across the globe. Starting his career on the PGA Tour of Australasia, he went on to a successful career on the European Tour before heading to the US to compete on the PGA Tour for nine years. O'Hern represented Australia at two World Cups and was a member of the International team at two Presidents Cups. He is the only man to have beaten Tiger Woods twice in the World Match Play Championship.

Acknowledgements

To my wife Alana, who's been with me from the beginning. She's seen it all: the highs, the lows, and everything in between. Thank you for inspiring me every day, my love. To Riley and Halle, who love making fun of their old man in the best possible way. Love you girls! To my parents for all their love and support over the years. To Neil Simpson, whose guidance took me from a pro who couldn't break 80 to being one of the most consistent players in the world, and to Neil McLean, who instilled in me the mental game foundations I built a career around. To James Williams, the best caddy and friend any player could ever want, and to Tony Bouffler for keeping me on the straight and narrow all these years. To the team at Hardie Grant Books – Pam Brewster for overseeing the project, Brooke Munday, Joanna Wong, and Michael Epis for all your hard work, and Sandy Grant for sharing my passion for golf and helping me bring this book to fruition.

Published in 2022 by Hardie Grant Books, an imprint of Hardie Grant Publishing

Hardie Grant Books (Melbourne)
Wurundjeri Country
Building 1, 658 Church Street
Richmond, Victoria 3121

Hardie Grant Books (London)
5th & 6th Floors
52–54 Southwark Street
London SE1 1UN

hardiegrantbooks.com

A catalogue record for this book is available from the National Library of Australia

How to Play Your Best Golf
ISBN 978 1 74379 804 1

10 9 8 7 6 5 4 3 2 1

Publisher: Pam Brewster
Project Editors: Joanna Wong and Brooke Munday
Editor: Michael Epis
Design Manager: Kristin Thomas
Designer: Murray Batten
Photography: Will Watt / Caddie magazine, Gary Lisbon, Nick O'Hern, Matt King / Stinger Getty Images, Harry How / Staff / Getty Images
Production Manager: Todd Rechner
Colour reproduction by Splitting Image Colour Studio
Printed in China by Leo Paper Products LTD.

Hardie Grant acknowledges the Traditional Owners of the country on which we work, the Wurundjeri people of the Kulin nation and the Gadigal people of the Eora nation, and recognises their continuing connection to the land, waters and culture. We pay our respects to their Elders past and present.